soul self

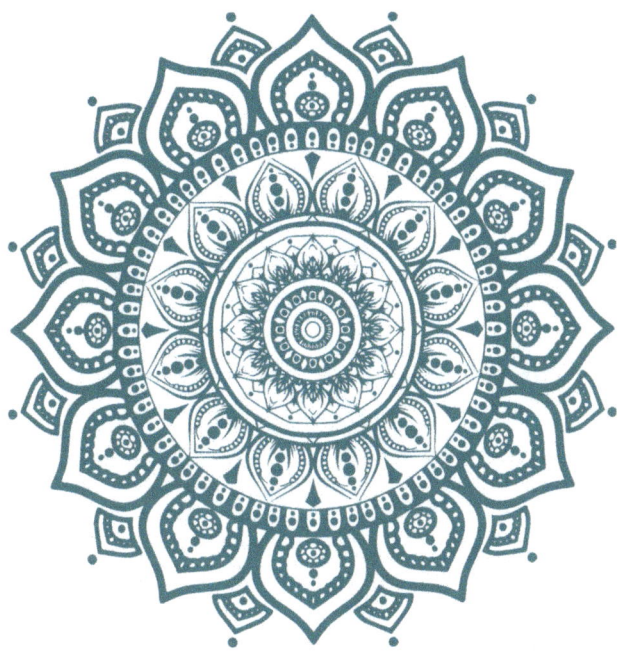

remember who you truly are;
embody your inner being &
shine your soul self on the world

alana clare power

Soul Self: Remember who you truly are, embody your inner being & shine your soul self on the world © Alana Clare Power 2023

The moral rights of Alana Clare Power to be identified as the author of this work have been asserted in accordance with the Copyright Act 1968.

ISBN 978-0-6458628-0-5

Any opinions expressed in this work are exclusively those of the author and are not necessarily the views held or endorsed by the Publisher.

All rights reserved. No part of this publication may be reproduced or transmitted by any means, electronic, photocopying or otherwise, without prior written permission of the author.

Disclaimer

All the information, techniques, skills and concepts contained within this publication are of the nature of general comment only, and are not in any way recommended as individual advice. The intent is to offer a variety of information to provide a wider range of choices now and in the future, recognising that we all have widely diverse circumstances and viewpoints. Should any reader choose to make use of the information herein, this is their decision, and the author and publisher/s do not assume any responsibilities whatsoever under any conditions or circumstances. The author does not take responsibility for the business, financial, personal or other success, results or fulfilment upon the reader's decision to use this information. It is recommended that the reader obtain their own independent advice.

dedication

This book is dedicated to my three children Jevaughn, Ceanais and Estelle. They inspire me daily as I watch them naturally gravitate towards being their authentic selves.

It is my hope for them that they will continue to be their original selves in every way and shine their light on the world in accordance with who they truly are.

"May all the children of the world know their true selves and may we hold the space for them to do so in every moment. May they shine their light of creation, expansion, and magnificence on the planet.

May they do this without distortion of any kind from another, without fear, coercion, pressure, manipulation, need, greed, or any other factor that pulls them towards another's agenda and away from their light.

May this be for all of us more often in our daily lives. May we know peace and love and be the light we have been looking for."

foreword

I have had the pleasure of knowing Alana for over a decade and throughout this time, have witnessed her personal journey in awe. Alana and I came together in 2010, with a common love of yoga and life. Her childlike essence and light-hearted nature and friendship have been such gifts. If there is one word to describe Alana, it would be authentic. She always shows up as her true soul self, and with that, has given others permission to feel comfortable in their own skin.

Alana has been a teacher and guide in many ways, both inside the yoga studio with her loyal tribe, and externally with family and friends. When times were tough, Alana has always looked for the light and found it and made positive choices for herself and her family. Her self-care extended to those around her, who have benefitted from her positive outlook on life.

If you have chosen to read this book, be prepared to discover more about yourself with little effort. Alana has this way with words. Her innate knowledge and wisdom will lead you to a deeper knowing, and once you tap in, you will find you will be able to reignite your light and reenergise from within. Her honest account and unique approach to life will bring comfort if you are also taking the road less travelled.

I have found Alana's book, Soul Self, has taken me on a deep journey within. Not only has this book been incredibly insightful, but her gentle instruction has also allowed me to self-reflect and feel more whole and well as a result.

Thank you for being a true friend and Soul Sista, Lana — you are an absolute superstar.

Julia Dyer
Communications Specialist, Marketing with Purpose

table of contents

Foreword vii
Preface 1
Meditation 5
Soul Self Meditation..7
The Energetic Chakra's 11
Life Lessons from the Chakra's 13
A Familiar Story... 16
Introduction... 19
Backstory... 25

Part 1: Remember...39
Remember Soul Deep... 41
Remember Soul Joy 49
Remember Soul Will 55
Remember Soul Love 63
Remember Soul Speak 69
Remember Soul Sees..77
Remember Soul Connect....................................... 83

Remember Soul Search 91

Part 2: Embody 103
Embody Soul Deep 105
Embody Soul Joy..121
Embody Soul Will... 125
Embody Soul Love 133
Embody Soul Speak 137
Embody Soul Sees..141
Embody Soul Connect 147
Embody Soul Search 151

Part 3: Shine 159
Shine Soul Deep...161
Shine Soul Joy 165
Shine Soul Will 169
Shine Soul Love 175
Shine Soul Speak 183
Shine Soul Sees... 189
Shine Soul Connect 195
Shine Soul Search 201
Conclusion 205
Questions and Answers with the Author 209
Acknowledgements 215
About the Author... 219

preface

"A candle loses nothing by lighting another candle."
JAMES KELLER

For as long as I can remember and to this day, I have been trying to figure out who I really am, why I'm really here, what the whole point or purpose of life on this planet is and so on. When you ask the questions for long enough, the answers generally start to find their way to you.

Soul Self may be a journey through the self, to the self and back again for you, the same journey I have been on and continue to be on, as I think the depths of who we are, why we're really here and any answers to this, can be endless.

This book has been partly birthed due to the overwhelming, overflowing content that weaves itself daily through me, to me and from me, like the type of content I could just imagine we all might carry deep within us. It's the type of stuff that your soul is bursting with and wishes it could say out loud but in daily life in our society your human self is perhaps scared and holds back due to fear of judgement, humiliation or worse, rejection.

It's the type of soul being content, that your inner child used to hear, but somewhere along the way stopped listening to its true self that once was the driving force.

For the majority of us, when we were young, we unconsciously started to listen to external voices from the people who surrounded us and that began to drown out our own innate inner voice. Eventually these outer voices became the programming that we'd operate from. If we ever heard the sweet sounds of our own true self in quiet moments, we would also likely be met with a programmed 'inner critic' or just other people's banter, which usually became imprinted throughout our childhood when we were at our most vulnerable and impressionable. Gradually this voice in our heads that played on repeat was the one we grew up with, grew into, and what we identified as, but this was not entirely who we truly were at our core.

This version of us that was not our full authentic self, represented us in many ways from how we acted, spoke, stood, behaved and so on. We picked up traits along the way that were not truly us, to the point where we lost who we were.

Our ego held on tight to these learned 'traits' in order to protect us. We grew fearful of speaking up at times when our authentic self would arise, for fear of being hurt or humiliated by others' judgements. We learned

preface

how and who to be, but it was not all of who we truly were. The adults that we are now, at times, may still hold back or speak from the inauthentic self, in order to stay safe in social situations that may seem threatening to our character or ego self.

Pain in our life is usually our biggest indicator that our soul is trying to wake us up in some way, trying to emerge like the beautiful butterfly that it is, but this can take some time. It is a process of unravelling and discovering who we are, sifting through the layers of who we are not and that can be downright scary sometimes to look within. We must be courageous and willing enough to trade the false self for who we actually are, if we seek to live a life with true purpose and honour our souls' mission in this life.

Thankfully, I have been on a mission to ignite my true self and overcome this fear of letting go of the false self. You see part of it was formed from our own ego to protect us when we needed it in order to survive. That is in the in the past now that we are adults and I believe in order to thrive it must die so we can shine.

I have not always been someone who speaks up and I know I do not do this in all aspects and all areas of my life just yet. For the most part and on reflection, I became very good at masking and being someone else who I thought would gain more approval from others. I also learnt how to be quite the sales lady and put on a persona that was not the real me. It may have been helpful in the past to survive in this world, but I am done with the art of surviving.

I prefer to be thriving and that involves being my authentic self at all costs because 'she' is who I am. It is a definite work in progress. When we are not in alignment with our true incredible being, it is usually due to fear or ego and when we are running on repeat of our conditioned programming. Most of us are not the exact embodiment of our inner beings just yet, but we are working on it.

The more we are able to be awake to who we truly are, the more we can shine our light fully as we feel the power of our being within and the support of the universe around us. We might also, by being our true selves, just stir something in someone else that has been dormant, asleep, or undisturbed, just as so too for ourselves it may have been.

So, it is my absolute pleasure to share with you my journey of allowing my authentic self to shine through: the highs and the lows, the years and the life lessons it has taken me to be my true self. It is my hope that I can be that one candle that lights up others.

meditation

The following meditation is one I have designed to allow you to drop into a space where you can begin to connect with your true self in a few ways.

Practice as many times as you need and notice each time how you deepen your connection with your authentic soul self. I always recommend a journal and a pen to write down your thoughts, experiences or things that come to you afterwards. Setting your surroundings up with some things that are personal and meaningful to you is also helpful to anchor in more of who you truly are. It could be an old childhood photograph of yourself, an ornament or crystal that connects you to more of your sense of self, some candles and incense is nice or whatever feels right for you.

Try to make sure you will be undisturbed for the duration of the meditation which can go from anywhere up to 10 minutes to as long as you'd like to stay in it. Also, unless you live in a hot climate you will need layers and blankets for warmth. Pillows or props like yoga blocks and bolsters are also helpful so you can comfortably sit or lie down for a good period of time.

The meditation is best listened to via audio. You may access this for free at www.alanaclarepower.com.au or alternatively make your own recording with your own voice on a personal device for your use only. This can be very powerful coming from yourself. You may also get a trusted friend to read it for you slowly as they hold space for you to do your meditation. After many practices it is my hope that you become so well versed in the meditation that you can guide yourself and drop into that connected soul self space more often. You will restore that true connection you once had the more time you spend with yourself on a deeper level.

Music can help you set the mood and connect in more with your soul. You will also no doubt have your own songs that can do this for you. However, meditation music is readily available on YouTube or Spotify and many other applications.

Music is a powerful tool to combine with soul connecting as it vibrates on a frequency that our souls can recognise. It's a great indicator for you, the music you are drawn to, what your soul loves, this is a window to your soul.

soul self meditation

*F*ind a quiet space where you will be undisturbed, lying down or seated. Closing down your eyes, begin by listening into the subtle sounds around you, both in the room and beyond. Move your awareness from sound to sound. Finally, listening to the sound of your own breathing and becoming aware of the breath at the nostrils...

Take a moment here...

Now begin to notice your whole physical body, start by noticing each limb, the arms and the legs including fingers and the toes, notice the torso, the back, neck, head, face, chest, navel and pelvic area. Become aware of the whole body in contact with the floor. Notice the beating of your own heart...

Take a moment here...

If your mind begins to wander at any stage, know this is normal in the beginning, just gently bring it back to focus on the practice without any judgement on yourself...

Take a moment here...

Notice any sensations you might be having in your body. Any areas that feel stiff, sore or tight. Try to breathe into those areas and relax them with the exhalation of the breath. Try to remain still, make small adjustments if you need in order to be comfortable...

Take a moment here...

Take three long and slow deep breaths. Feel yourself letting go and the earth beneath you supporting you. As you breathe in, feel the weight of the body on the floor and as you breathe out, feel the body becoming lighter...

Take a moment here...

Become aware of your breath at the nostrils, the coolness on the inhalation and warmth on the exhalation. Notice the different smells around you in the room.

Become aware of the taste in your mouth at the moment.

Notice the warmth of the body that is covered by clothing and the coolness on the skin that is not covered.

Now notice the space behind the closed eyes. You may see colour or light or just an inky darkness.

Take a moment here...

Now become aware of the mental chatter inside your head. Stay there a while not getting involved but being the observer of your thoughts. Sit for a bit longer, ignore the mental chatter, hear just the silence and subtle sounds around you...

Take a moment here...

Now listen for a different voice inside you, trying always to speak to you amongst the busyness of your mind and life all around you. There it is, in that feeling, that subtle knowing that becomes strong, feels powerful and begins to lead the way.

While the mental chatter gets softer, the inner voice gets louder, and before you know it, you have an awareness of something new and in fact it is a remembering of something that has been with you all along. It feels somehow familiar, comforting, supportive. It may feel like 'home' to you. It is not your judging mind, daily thoughts but something more powerful.

This essence, that is you. An essence that is love. Something that can not be measured, touched or taken away. This is your connection to source, god or whatever you perceive it to be and it is through this connection you will discover you...

Take some time here...

Linger here as you discern between thoughts in your mind that will try and pop up and your inner voice.

Listen, feel and stay with your inner self. What are you noticing? Who is the one who is noticing? You have become the observer of your thoughts, the observer *of your human self, you are tapped into your soul self, your souls source.*

You may stay here as long as you are comfortable to do so...

When you are ready to come out of the meditation take your time. Feel into the connection between the body and the floor. Remember the room that you are in.

The four walls, the ceiling and the floor. Bring the awareness to the breath at the nostrils and slowly begin to open your eyes. Become familiar again with your surrounds.

Take some time here for yourself...

Stretch your body however feels good and right for you. Sit with your experience in silence and feel free to write anything down. You may return to this practice at anytime.

the energetic chakra's

Whilst writing this book I started to notice a synergy between the pieces I was writing and the energetic chakra system. As you read through the pages if you are aware of the chakras, you may notice the chapters tend towards correlating with this system. You may blissfully go ahead and read through this book and be none the wiser. Either is fine and perfect, however, I have offered an extended understanding of the relationship between life and our own energetic system. Below is a piece I wrote for the Extraordinary Life Magazine produced by Emily Gowor who is an inspirational writer, author and keynote speaker. The article is on life lessons from the chakras, giving you a basic understanding on the chakras and the interplay between them and our existence with life.

It's also been a beautiful way to express how the soul and its interplay with the energetic body is at the seat of all we do. Just like the soul is a witness to the physical body and all it might go through, so too is it a witness to life's effects on our energetic chakra system.

The more knowledge and the more awareness we have on the different layers, bodies and systems we have, the more empowered we are to heal our bodies and minds so that we may be the best versions of ourselves in this life. To me, the chakra system can bring some order to seemingly disorder in life by acting as a balancing tool and guidance system to support us along our journey.

life lessons from the chakra's

The wisdom of the energetic chakra's can be a tool for growth and change.

The chakras are a spinning vortex or wheel of light. They are the junctions that manage the flow of life force that runs through the energy body. Tuned into our life and life force energy, these energetic wheels of insight mirror back to us our current state, situation or flow in life.

Depletions, excess or blockages of these energy centers can manifest in our mental, emotional and physical bodies and even affect our connection to the spirit world. Further than that, they hold much wisdom relating to life lessons that we all can benefit from.

When we are facing certain challenges in life, are feeling unmotivated or uninspired, chances are some of our chakras may be out of balance. Like a feedback system, specific chakras carry a myriad of information. For example, they can tell us areas where we may be pushing too hard or why we are feeling stuck.

The chakras can help us reflect on the many personal aspects of our life. This is where the life lessons can come in and we can work to improve and grow in those areas, hence mastering those attributes. The seven main chakra points and some examples of associated attributes with the relevant life lessons are as follows.

The **Base Chakra** can be associated with stability, security and self-sufficiency.

We can learn that taking responsibility for ourselves, for our basic needs, selfcare and even financial stability can lead to our physical wellbeing as well as feeling grounded and secure in life.

The **Sacral Chakra** can be associated with our joy, creation and sexuality. Here we can learn that looking after ourselves by allowing more joy into our lives, quite possibly through creative pursuits, can give a us a sense of feeling good in life and open to changes.

The **Solar Plexus Chakra** can be associated with self-confidence, self-worth and personal power. We can learn in this area about setting boundaries with our time and energy as well as living an authentic life on our terms, leading to feeling in our power, feeling self-confident with who we are and worthy of pursuing our dreams.

The **Heart Chakra** can be associated with love, compassion and forgiveness.

When we are able to love unconditionally, we can have compassion, understanding and find it easier to forgive ourselves and others.

The **Throat Chakra** can be associated with communication, expression and personal truth. The life lesson here is to speak up, speak your truth and express and articulate yourself clearly and authentically.

The **Third Eye Chakra** can be associated with Intuition, instincts and a higher knowing. Life lessons here can be around trusting your gut feeling, listening to or trusting the feelings you are getting even on a vibrational level. Trusting your inner knowing.

The **Crown Chakra** can be associated with divine, spirit connection and a oneness with all. Life lessons here can be around our mental health as well as knowledge and spiritual enlightenment.

There are many resources available and ways in which you can work with the chakras. For example, through meditation, visualization, breathwork, sound vibration and even intuition. A trained energy practitioner can give your chakra points a tune up and cleanse, as well as bring the energy back into balance.

By understanding the power of the chakras, you can raise your awareness of the potential impacts on different areas of your life and heal. Once we're tuned in, we can tune up our energy. We can reflect on and use these lessons from the chakras to master our life.

a familiar story

"ONCE UPON A TIME...There was a bright beam of light coming from inside a tiny clear crystal white egg. It lay on a leaf under the moonlight, just like in the children's book called 'The Very Hungry Caterpillar' by Eric Carle.

By morning just before the sun rose, a tiny creature crawled its way out of a small crack in the egg and out popped a very tiny human.

As the tiny human grew up it consumed everything around it from food to everything in its environment. The tiny human absorbed everything it heard, watched, and experienced throughout life until it became all of those things.

As the tiny human grew older through many sunrises and sunsets, it went on a very big journey. The roads were winding and bumpy and sometimes scary, even confusing. One day the big human found itself completely lost. It forgot where home was and had a big headache, so it decided to rest. It was cold so it made itself a shelter that looked a bit like a cocoon.

Inside the shelter it was warm, quiet, dark, and cosy. The big human started to remember what life was once like as a tiny human. A smile grew on its face but then there was also sadness, for the big human had forgotten who it truly was and why it was in fact here on this planet Earth.

The big human stayed in its shelter for many years, spending time doing things its heart wanted to, as its brain had become too tired from life.

One day when the big human was doing what it loved, it heard someone speak.

No one was there of course as the big human was all alone in its shelter. It heard it again and again and again and it began to recognise the voice. It remembered it had once heard that voice inside the tiny egg and when it was a very tiny human. The voice was the tiny human's soul self, seemingly speaking to the tiny human.

It had been so long that the two rejoiced like old friends that hadn't seen each other for a very, very, long time.

The big human's eyes grew wide, its skin glowed, and it had an energy that could jump a million miles. The big human had found its true self once again and its headache went away and its mind relaxed. Its heart grew full and began to be led by the inner voice it had heard. There was no more confusion . The big human was not lost; it had found its true self, the road home, and its way forward and never felt alone in the world again.

The big human grew older and lived a wonderful life doing everything its soul had ever wanted to on planet Earth. It created magic on Earth for many more humans to come and enjoy its magnificent soul print that it left after it flew away as the most beautiful butterfly ever seen. It turned out that it was the heart that was the gateway to the soul self and that the soul self is the true superpower here on Earth waiting for the human to take the lead with the soul in the driver's seat.

THE END..."

introduction

Sometimes, just like in the life cycle of a butterfly, we too go through a process of becoming. We start out as a pure soul, become this physical human being, and take on and accumulate what surrounds us. If we are fortunate enough in this life, we go through the process of transformation over and over again. What evolves is us being able to live in the highest version of ourselves possible at any one time. This allows us to uplift the world around us with our everincreasing vibration and leave a positive impact on the planet.

"People talk about caterpillars becoming butterflies as though they just go into a cocoon, slap on wings, and are good to go. Caterpillars have to dissolve into a disgusting pile of goo to become butterflies. So if you're a mess wrapped up in blankets right now, keep going."

— JENNIFER WRIGHT

Many of us throughout a lot of our lives don't really take the time out to discover or remember who we truly are. We're caught up in the web of life since the day we are born. We're overstimulated by our modern surroundings, influenced and conditioned right from birth. If our spirit within is strong and determined to execute its life's contract and purpose here on Earth, it will continually pursue its goals and try to push through like a butterfly trying to come out of its cocoon.

This transformation can manifest in many ways. The process may even begin as an illness, seen as a disorder of some type, with us feeling lost, confused, disconnected perhaps. I can tell you it is all part of the process. A butterfly coming out of its cocoon is pretty messy and requires persistence, courage, strength and to hold its own as it tries to integrate its beautiful self with the world. As it stretches its wings and professes to the world its beauty and who it came here to be, it will be met with life itself or should I say life will be met with it, as its highest version.

Take the life cycle of a butterfly: it is first laid as an egg, grows into a caterpillar, and takes in all of life. When it's time, the caterpillar builds its cocoon and goes through transformation. It embodies its highest form, what it truly came here to be. It then emerges from the chrysalis and shines bright as a brilliant butterfly. We too can go through this process in life to remember, embody, and shine the way our soul intended.

"We are all born free and spend a lifetime becoming slaves to our own false truths."

AUTHOR UNKNOWN

introduction

When we connect to our true self, we feel light, joyous, and unstoppable, ready to conquer the world with our love and our passion for life. That's how powerful our true self really is.

We are here to remember the authentic self within the self, to embody, to embrace, all of who we are. We are not here to hide, not here to run from the complete self that lies within, the self that we sometimes can't ever recall meeting. The self that we may see glimpses of in our quiet moments, but then perhaps we find our programmed mind or ego, quickly assuming the role of who we are instead when it's time to integrate with our modern lives.

Like an imposter and without us even realising, this manifestation of programming begins to run on repeat. It becomes who we are on the outside and our whole lives risk being led by this false identity. The world around us often supports this false identity as it assimilates cooperatively with society and the rules and regulations we find around us.

The world approves of who this identity is and so it gets stronger and stronger and louder and louder until we can't even hear our true self anymore. Our false identity doesn't often speak our truth and quietly shuts its mouth at the appropriate times. It learns to keep you safe by suggesting in your thoughts that you blend into the background where nobody will notice you. This false imposter doesn't like risk and will fill you with fear or illusion every time it thinks you need protecting. It is formed in childhood when you are at your most vulnerable and impressionable. The ego often finds many reasons to try to be your boss. A healthy ego can be helpful but not if it's out of balance.

Thankfully there is hope; we can wake up from this robot-run life and remember who we truly are. We can nurture that voice within until it is strengthened and lights your way once again, as it did when you were first born into this world. Your soul self is waiting to be realised and wanting to be set free on Earth. Within these pages, I hope you find the key that unlocks your soul, and walk right through that door.

Soul Self will take you on a journey of self-reflection, a remembering and true knowing of who you really are at a soul level. Through my own journey and experiences in life I will offer insights and ways in which this can be done.

There are many tools in life we can access to know our true self and through these tools we can start to remember our inner essence and our soul print and be reunited with the brilliant being within.

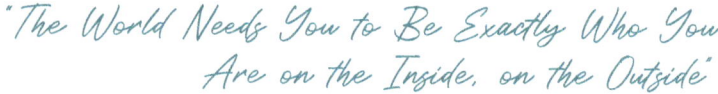

"The World Needs You to Be Exactly Who You Are on the Inside, on the Outside"

Soul Self will share wisdom to show you ways in which you can embody your being once you remember who you truly are. Somewhere along the way most of us forget who we are, but if we are fortunate, we have what some may call an awakening that leads us on our path of transformation. Soul Self is about guiding you through yourself to yourself and then bringing out the authentic you. It's about reawakening, remembering who you truly are and then embodying and living the way your soul intended.

Join me on a journey as I share with you my experiences of my own soul ignition. Remember how to know and love who you truly are and develop an awareness of the soul self, the self that lies beneath the surface. Gain the courage to be able to stand strong in your authenticity with grace and especially when faced with adversity from the outside world. Enhance the quality of your life and your relationships simply by embodying your true self that's on the inside, on the outside.

Discover how to truly come home to the self, ways in which to do that and how to stay on that journey. This is so important in order to live the life your soul intended to and so important not only for the self, but for all of humanity and our planet.

The book will help you understand how being your true self not only raises your vibration, but that of the human collective. The world so desperately needs this if we are to transform a world from bleak to bliss, from madness to magic, and from weariness to wonderful.

Call me a dreamer, maybe, but I know our infinite potential because I've seen my own and many others bring theirs to the surface. That which is in me and in others is also in you. We are not separate on a soul level; in that sense, we are all one and from the same source. You are not here by chance. You are part of all creation: it's time to find your shine.

This is not just a bunch of words on a page laced with hope, but a sure knowing that the light that is within me is also in you. Shine!

backstory

"God changes caterpillars into butterflies, sand into pearls and coal into diamonds using time and pressure. He is working on you too."

RICK WARREN

"Being A Young Caterpillar"

It was 2008 and I had a young baby girl (about 8 months old) and a 4-year-old boy full of energy but also with many quirks and sensitivities. Unbeknownst to me, there were some real good reasons why my little boy would melt down more than a dozen times throughout the day. We'd go for a walk to get said sister to sleep in the pram and if it was windy, he would scream and drop his body to the ground. Sister would scream from the commotion as you might imagine and this wouldn't really induce relaxing sleeping conditions, even though the sea breeze might normally allow a person to nod off on an otherwise pleasant day.

Life was hectic to say the least; we had just moved to a new area, I was a fairly young mum by today's standards (then 28 years old) of a new baby and a preschooler who was having some health challenges. Later we would discover through formal assessment, his autism. He also had had a diagnosis of epilepsy since seizures occurred from just 9 months of age.

Hubby was gone 12 hours a day working a job in the city for the sole purpose of tackling piling up financial burdens (he wasn't doing inspired, purposeful work just yet) and I was feeling fairly alone in a new area as I'm sure many new mothers can relate to, juggling small children and home life.

Prior to having my son, first born, at 24 years old, I had had a short career and business of my own which included travelling overseas and importing gifts and homewares after working for an importer. I left this life of ambition and inspiration to do what you do when you supposedly 'grow up' and become responsible, or so I thought. In other words, get married (although that part was for love and still is to this day, I feel very blessed), buy a house (aka get a mortgage), get a 'stable' job, and start a family.

All this just short of turning 25 years old. Did it make me happy? If you are reading this book, I bet you already know the answer to that question. However, it's what society taught us, what our parents and people who 'cared' about us taught us. It's what our parents and parents' parents did. This was life, right? You should be happy, right? You find the 'one' and live happily ever after? Well, my soul was certainly searching for more; through my soul's whispers I knew there was a greater purpose for me to follow. There was more to my journey yet to unfold that would guide me in getting closer to who I truly was.

You can either drown in the hardship, your past or present trauma and the heaviness of life, or you can take a breath (sometimes many are required), a step back, the weight off for a moment and remember who you truly are.

Remember why you came here.

This didn't truly come for me until much later when I dove deeply into reconnecting with my heart and soul in 2014 through my intensive yoga teacher training.

"A Caterpillar – The Next Stage"

Beyond that, I began embodying more of my true self and set the wheels in motion around 2018. With a breath of fresh air and a real sense of freedom, that year as a family we truly 'unplugged' from the matrix we call life and went on our camping trip for a year together in a tent.

Prior to that, in 2017, I had completed and attended a course and retreats on deeply embodying my unique gifts and purpose, more deep soul work that would bring me even closer to my true self.

On reflection, my soul has always been wanting to surface and it's incredible the people, places, and things we energetically call into our lives in order to do so. I remember being about 4 years old and my mother taking me to the yoga ashram for the weekend. It was my first immersion into meditation and where I first distinguished between my physical body, mind, and soul.

After that, I was about 18 when I next attended my mother's yoga class and beyond that, was very interested in more deeply exploring the soul within. Around the same age I attended a soul deep self-development workshop called 'Born to be Free' and obtained a pranic energy healing certification. I would continue on that exploratory soul journey back to myself in various ways and through different modalities right up until the present day.

I had come to realise over this time how much society, or the system rather, has us 'plugged' into a regime that works to keep people in some kind of order, when in truth, the way western society is set up, really can become part of people's private struggles and personal chaos. It can also cause some people's sickness, depression, anxiety, and stress.

More than ever, and now as I write this in 2022, I feel this fast paced, unnatural, capitalist focused way of life that increases pressure on families with longer work days, nose to the grind so to speak has a detrimental effect on our children and their health. It can effect children as young as five years old, not to mention younger, as they are born into a world where it is encouraged to live an existence further from the soul, nature and natural paces than ever before. As humans, we are nature and our bodies and spirits can't thrive at that pace; we are not robots, yet we seem to be heading into a robotic world.

"You Get to the Point Where You Outgrow Your Current Skin"

We sold our house in 2017, bought a large tent, swapped our cars for a JEEP and went camping up the east coast of Australia with our three children then aged 5, 10, and 13 years old. What an amazing year and adventure as we allowed our bodies to unwind to the rhythms of life and slow down to a pace that put smiles back on our faces and sunshine in our steps.

For 11 months we camped in a tent with only a few stays in luxury apartments or other accommodation as a treat. I said goodbye to friends and family, to the house, the car, my work (then running my own small yoga business) and even our beloved dalmatian. We threw caution to the wind as they say and set off on an adventure led only by the sunshine, our sense of adventure, and wherever our hearts were called to. This process of growth is one we continue to go through over and over. In fact, the caterpillar outgrows and sheds its skin over five times before it builds its chrysalis.

"It Is Necessary to Spend Some Time In Your Cocoon"

Since then, the past almost four years we have put our focus towards what brings true meaning in our lives . We have begun creative projects left, right and centre as we follow our souls' callings and not the calling of what society or anybody else might want us to do. To some, yes, we are real 'alternatives', hippies, nomads, whatever you might want to call us. To us we are just following our souls' callings, inviting in creativity, and living life on our terms.

We are allowing our lives to unfold naturally and organically as we put one foot in front of the other, tuning into a soul led path.

For me, family life itself has had a large part in steering my ship in doing what I do today. In digging deep and finding stillness, to find the gifts and what I'm truly passionate about.

Quite often, we, over the years, would try to work away from the home but found that our children's needs were always calling us back. Not realising at the time that all three of our children would be diagnosed as being on the autism spectrum which I now understand as being neurodivergent. For them, assimilating with normal life, going to school, and just general daily living can be a challenge. At times when I or my husband were trying to build a career outside of the home this would become our challenge too. We found ourselves being pulled to care for our children at home, beyond normal parenting requirements, even as they grew into older children and teens.

As blessings in disguise come, not so obvious to begin with, we eventually surrendered to this need of our children requiring more and more support as they got older from us at home. We have since created a life together as a family that supports their needs and allows us to work around them from home whilst they grow and learn in a home school setting or whatever work/study requirements they may have at the time that may need our support.

More than ever, this has given them and us flexibility, it allows them and us to work at our own pace, set our own timetable and be drawn to what we truly love, naturally, without too much pressure of external forces.

A more balanced and happy family life, freedom from external stress, and freedom to choose what we want to pursue whilst being there to support and encourage each other along the way has been the result. At the end of the day when your soul is not happy, it will push through, view what is happening as chaos or not working for you in life and ask that you make the changes. Are you listening to your soul's callings and how might life be trying to steer you in the direction of your true purpose?

Turning your ship around sometimes requires that you listen to the messages that are being thrown your way which often come as challenging situations waiting for you to rise above with a solution. Turning your ship around requires you to get out of your own way by not continuing to bang your head against that same brick wall.

It never happens in a moment but in many moments, years even and dedication to pursue what your soul came here to do. There are many lessons to learn, and I don't have all the answers for you, but I can tell you that you certainly do on the inside. I can show you how and where to look, how I've steered my ship and took notice of what life was presenting me with at the time and importantly followed my souls urges.

Most importantly, gotten out of my own way by listening to my inner guidance system. Has it been easy? No. Especially when I don't listen to the signs (that's when the hard lessons come) and even when I do, listening and embodying takes courage. It's not always the easy road; in fact, it requires me at times to go off the beaten track! It requires me to do things differently, move out of my comfort zone, grow and strengthen and expect that a lot of close family and friends may think I have gone crazy! It is usually just fear, as I'm sure they care very much about me; however, I always remember this is not my fear to take on.

What was in front of me may have looked like chaos, trauma, drama, financial hardship, or relationship turmoil. As it turns out, it has actually been my ticket to getting on my path. When things are not okay in life, I do something about it; it can be that simple. I mean actually do something about it, look at it, recognise it for what it truly is as opposed to drown it out with unhealthy habits or addictions and continue on a destructive path rather than embrace that my problems are there for me to see through to the other side.

At times in my life, I have unconsciously chosen unhealthy habits, like partying too hard with girlfriends on weekends in the past. I would drown my sorrows with too many drinks at the bar and numb out any sadness. Don't get me wrong; there is nothing wrong with going out with friends, dancing, and having a good time, but it's a problem when limits go over board and it becomes an unhealthy way of life instead of a healthy outlet.

These days, I tend to sit around with girlfriends drinking tea and pulling tarot cards, laughing until we cry munching on good, healthy food. I still like to dance and sing but this is mostly in my lounge room or in the kitchen when it's time to create dinner!

Choosing a healthier lifestyle for myself has also been a part of listening to my true soul's callings. We also get to an age where we really have to listen to our body or suffer the consequences. I think when we are younger, we take our health for granted; as we age this is just not possible. This is also a part of the process in waking up to who we truly are. Honouring our body temple and giving it what it needs more of the time rather than what we think we might want.

Finding new ways to satisfy our life's cravings and finding a healthier option for longevity, vitality and thriving, is an important part of not just growing up but growing close to our authentic self. We always want the best for ourselves; we can just sometimes get caught up in unhealthy human coping mechanisms. The same can be said for unhealthy relationships we might keep or not truly giving ourselves the life we deserve.

So, the past few years have been spent listening to the callings of my soul because she knows the way. I have a dedicated yoga room for that with a lock on the door. The shower or toilet is also good for downloading inspiration and listening to the song of your soul so you can dance to the beat of it! A walk alone will also do it; in fact, there is no end to activities, places and spaces that will allow you to listen to your soul speak, but you need to be alone, that is the key! It could be on the train or plane or in your car, upon waking in the morning or last thing at night. If you ask, wait and listen; it will come.

"Becoming a Butterfly"

So back to what I was viewing as chaos and drama in my life which was really the power of the soul pushing through! It was happening to me and to my family around me, my husband and children. All of our souls pushing through to be here can come across as hectic and dramatic when it's all at the same time! I guess you could say for my family it was a domino effect. When one person shines his or her light, it gives the other person permission to do so and his or her soul gets restless until it's heard.

After travelling, we settled back in country Victoria in Ballarat, out of busy Melbourne. My girls started at a very small primary school and my son at a larger high school. Hubby and I began to bring our dream of building a tiny house into reality and so we went on with life but in a slightly different way. I didn't return to yoga teaching because if I'm honest I felt burnt out after throwing myself into a three-year near solo yoga business straight from teacher training. I wanted some time for me, to integrate everything thus far. I also felt called to explore something new and many things have unfolded since.

Currently I spend my weekdays working on this book and my writing pursuits whilst guiding my children to follow their hearts and passions. After a year or so back in school my girls quickly decided it wasn't for them and that activity-based learning for their creative and artistic pursuits was the way forward along with other extracurricular activities woven in. All doors are always open for any direction they choose to go in, for all three of my children.

My husband is also following his calling and passions getting back into doing what he loves, designing and crafting unique pieces of furniture that is more like functional pieces of art works. I couldn't be happier and couldn't ask for more right now as we work to pursue businesses that are close to our hearts and in alignment with our callings and why we are here.

There is no one giant step, no great leap or bound, just a gentle steering of your ship moment to moment that steers you on and keeps you on your path as you follow the stars and what's written in your heart. Listen to your soul's calling as you dare to quieten the noise around you telling you what's important.

"And every day, the world will drag you by the hand, yelling, "This is important! And this is important! You need to worry about this! And this! And this!" And each day it is up to you to yank your hand back, put it on your heart and say, "No, this is what's important!" -
Ian Thomas

What's important is that you come here and live the life you are designed for! Shift the consciousness of this planet by being the inspired human you are with your soul as your engine. Are you ready for your soul's ignition? It's ready when you are.

"The thing is this, if we don't wake up to who we are, we will fall asleep to who we are not. We will live but we will not be truly alive."

AUTHOR UNKNOWN

part 1
remember

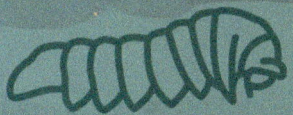

To Truly Know Yourself, Is to Truly Love Who You Are

What does it mean to remember?

1. *Have in or be able to bring to one's mind an awareness of (someone or something from the past) – Oxford Dictionary*

To remember who you are is to look for that person that was always you, the original you. It's to search within yourself and remember the pure essence, the being you incarnated as, the one who once was, before you took on your human identity that formed around you as a result of life itself and as a result of your environment, influences, and importantly the subconscious mind.

chapter 1
remember soul deep

"Life is a school, where you learn how to remember what your soul already knows."

AUTHOR UNKNOWN

Who We Truly Are

It's a big question, one we usually skip over in the hustle and bustle of life until the universe decides for us it's time to take a look. If it gets to the universe deciding, this usually happens when we least expect it and can come in the form of a harder lesson. That is, unless we've been open to listening each day and are taking some time out to come back to the self, come home to our creator, God or source.

They say we have free will here on this planet and I believe that to be true, but I also believe we came committed to a purpose, signed a contract and have much work to do here. Both teaching and learning, evolving and growing and lifting the vibration of Earth. That's me anyhow and we are all different. We all play a different part in the symphony of life, and we are all important in the greater plan. It's not all work and no play though, that would be joyless, right? I believe we are here to create, bring our true essence to life, remember all the vibrant colours that our soul has to offer and individually but collectively create a beautiful world.

So how can we possibly create if we don't truly know the creator? Most of us are born seeing what's on the outside and never taught about what's on the inside. Worse still, we are taught to silence our inner voice, learn what is expected and become a robot of society's imprints instead of being free to explore and be the magical being that we are within. We are true miracles, and the biggest tragedy is never allowing the soul to come to light but instead living below the surface, never truly allowing it to step into the physical form and shine.

Your job is to listen, trust and believe that the world needs you to be exactly who you are on the inside, on the outside. This is ultimately your purpose, to be the true you. The universe is rooting for you. It's rooting for you every time you get brave enough to say what's really on your mind, set your boundaries in that toxic relationship or begin that new business you've been dreaming of.

It's rooting for you when you don't let fear stand in your way or the ego trick you into not doing what you've always wanted and telling you to be safe instead. That universe (God, source, our creator or whatever it is you believe) is waiting for you to be the authentic being that you are and it will always have your back when you follow your soul's guidance, your heart, your path, your callings. It is universal law and when we trust that, life blooms.

How do we know the difference between the inner voice and the outer voice?

Usually, the outer voice is the loud and noisy chatter in your head that worries, thinks the worst and is mostly on repeat. Your inner voice (true self) is very quiet and comes from the heart space up to the mind only to articulate or find words to express itself out through your mouth. It may be that it finds itself expressed through your fingertips if you are a writer for example, or by building something if you are creative in that way. Your natural gifts are directly related to who you truly are and what you came here to do.

Your soul self is the creative, brilliant, spontaneous steady flow that is very sure of itself and never questions itself. If you find yourself overthinking, doubting or in fear that's not your inner voice. The inner voice is pure love, flowing energy, and excitement. Its opponent can be the ego, since the ego is designed to keep you safe; however, your inner voice is pure love and the very essence of you only wanting good things for you. Your inner voice wants you to reach your potential and your highest good whilst you are journeying here on Earth.

There is nothing wrong with a healthy ego; it's just when it becomes overinflated or out of balance that problems can arise.

Pausing to Remember You

This may come as a short and sweet message, but it is most likely the biggest piece of advice I could possibly give. It is essential to take time out, alone, in total peace - even if it's 10 minutes per day - to stay close to who you truly are. I have a dedicated yoga room for this but a good set of earphones with some relaxing music along with closed eyes and a big 'do not disturb' sign can also work wonders. Failing that, a walk by yourself marvelling at nature will also bring you back home to the self.

How noisy life can be, and we can easily forget who we are. We forget the wondrous being that came here and the connection we have with all of life including the subtle energies that surround us, the energetic connection that is the web of life. Take some time to relax back into you and operate from that soul self: it's who you truly are. Getting out into nature is even better: watching a sunrise or sunset, staring at a moonlit night sky, watching water flow, and reconnecting with the elements to bring you back to your natural self.

Knowing and Aligning With Your Soul Self

Knowing, developing, and maintaining a relationship with our soul self is the key to be able to come into alignment with who we truly are. Our purpose and path in life may be found simply through doing this. There are many modalities, healers, psychics, and guides we can access here on Earth to help us do this; however, the knowledge is all within us.

Most times when I access different modalities it comes as a confirmation to what I thought was my purpose or my truth. It shows me that I once knew and still hold that sacred knowledge within me. I am here to tell you that you can access that wisdom through you, just by being connected to your soul self. Your purpose is to be who you truly are and through that you will be guided along the path your soul wants to walk in this lifetime and the lessons it wishes to learn, the experiences it chooses to have, and the life it came to lead.

Whenever I am out of alignment, I either notice and take the initiative to take time out, access my chosen modalities for support, or be booted by the universe. The latter is never so pleasant and can consist of chaos, break downs, overwhelm or illness until I listen and heed the signs and messages.

Many times, I have tried to walk away from my purpose for it just seemed easier to live a simple quiet earthly life with my family, bury my head and not show up. It feels comfortable for a while, until it doesn't. It's likened to lying in bed on a cold morning with the bed warmer turned up high instead of getting up. It's only going to feel so good for so long until you get thirsty or need the bathroom or get bored or your body begins to ache from lack of movement. I believe we can only sit for so long, hide out for a time or be off track for a little while, until we start to get these reminders from the universe. The universe says, 'I'm going to keep you on track' and it does! Don't hate it; thank it. It's in alignment with your soul's calling.

Your soul self is in alignment with the universe. Sometimes it's just waiting for the human version to catch up or get back on track. Whilst we do have free will as humans on this Earth, we also have soul contracts and I believe one way or another, the universe will always help you out to fulfil yours. It may not always appear that way; however, look for the lesson or the message in the madness. Somehow it's always nudging us towards our path when we are veering off.

Take notice of the signs and don't be afraid to be drawn to whatever healing modalities will best serve you and guide you on your path. Sometimes it's a great teacher, mentor, or your own soul self that you tap into and sometimes it's seeking others to assist in your journey. Whatever it is, it is lifelong that we may need guidance if we are to stay on track, live in alignment, and fulfil our purpose, our soul reason for being here. At the very least, accessing that guidance from our soul self or perhaps with assistance from others, there are so many modalities that can serve this specific purpose.

There is so much guidance that can tell you about you or confirm, I should say, as I truly believe we already hold that knowledge within. Embodiment tools in Chapter 9 will share with you a handful of what I know, what I've experienced, and what has helped me in times of need. All of these things are tools to assist with knowing and aligning and becoming the embodiment of your soul self.

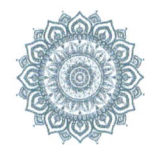

chapter 2
remember soul joy

"I can remember the joy that I came to this Earth for."

AUTHOR UNKNOWN

The Joy of Being You

The world needs you to be exactly who you are on the inside, on the outside.

The world needs the joy of being you, the freedom and the peace that comes with being able to live in this world and be yourself. That is undeniable freedom within: to be able to be you, to not need to fit into somebody else's system, somebody else's world and somebody else's creation of how to live.

We all come to this world, even identical twins, as unique beings. There are no two beings, butterflies, birds, flowers, or anything, not even two vegetables, that are exactly the same. This is because everything is created in one split moment, one split second of each other. Even with twins, where the egg splits at the same time, even if they become identical in looks, the way they might speak or any other factor, will still have differences. We are all a focal point of difference in this world and that focal point is collective consciousness becoming aware of itself. In every single moment, we are becoming aware, consciousness is becoming aware of itself, of the experiences that we experience in this world. The world needs you to be exactly who you are on the inside, on the outside, so we can realise the true tapestry of life that is to be.

We can construct or create that into form to the naked eye of any living being, animal or plant on this Earth. If consciousness is to become aware of its true self fully, we need to allow ourselves to be fully who we are. Only then will we realise who we are, the truth of who we truly are together as one consciousness, evolving continuously and bringing that into physical creation.

When we stop and gain an insight into who we really are, we will realise how much joy there is within. When we continually come back home to ourselves, come back home to who we truly are, and, most importantly, know how to get there, we understand we are joy. Knowing how to come home to the self, knowing what your true self is and being able to, step by step, start to bring out who you really are into the physical world is to remember the joy within. It is to remember the unique being that you are but know you are from a collective source or energy that is essentially available and connected to all of us. This brings a lighter way of looking at the world, a peace and a feeling of joy.

The Playful Child Within

When was the last time you allowed yourself some joy? When was the last time you put your schedule down just to dance, sing, create or do whatever the child within or your soul self was calling to do? When was the last time you allowed yourself to be silly, play games, or have some good old-fashioned fun?

When did we start caring too much what other people think and lose that child-like part of us that wants to just have fun? Yes, you can be old and let your hair down; you are never too old to have some fun. The best part is now that you are an adult you don't even need anyone's permission! Yet we place restrictions on our own inner child due to the conditioning of our world around us as we grew up. Always hearing stop being silly, don't do that, sit still at the table and the list goes on.

I have to catch my serious adult self when I'm 'parenting' my own children. Whilst we need boundaries, we also need freedom to be ourselves and just have fun! This is the joyful part of letting our true selves shine, allowing our beautiful colours to be seen on the outside! Imagine all your beautiful colours hidden within, for no one else to see - or very few - for fear of judgement. Imagine a book cover was left blank, dull, and boring but on the inside the book was bursting with wisdom, knowledge, value, and joy! Wouldn't it be sad that people would just walk on by not having any idea of the magic that's within? Isn't it time to let that spill out of you? God knows we need it in our world more than ever. Go on! I dare you; shine bright like a beautiful rainbow butterfly; show us all your colours! Brighten up this world with your big, bold, and beautiful self.

A Stable Foundation

To be your true self in the world it is important to not only know who you truly are but have your feet planted firmly in the foundations of your true self. Like a tree swaying in the wind, you want those roots to run deep. More to the point, you want to be connected deeply to the root of who you are. "Don't should on me" was a term I heard in my 30s when a friend invited me along to a workshop.

The basis of this that comes to mind now is that anything that is swaying you or pulling you from being your true self is not for you. Anything that is not aligned with who you truly are is not your path. I have gotten very good at saying 'NO' these days and not feeling guilty about it. I no longer feel like I need to take on other people's projections, thoughts, feelings, ideals, or judgements.

Nobody knows you better than your own soul does and it's the only voice to tell you 'should' in my opinion. Being firm about who you are and standing strong with awareness of that in your everyday life will see you living a life exactly as your soul intended. This is the foundation for your authentic life to grow and soon you will blossom and bloom into the beautiful being you were always meant to be. For a lot of us we must unlearn the conditioning and swaying that took us away from who we truly are. It is a healing journey before it is an easy swim to living a life of abundance and joy, doing and being exactly what you came here for.

chapter 3
remember soul will

"Remember that your will and divine will are one. When the two are in alignment you are in your truest power."

AUTHOR UNKNOWN

You at Your Core

You can re-write your life, chase your dreams, feel better, think better, be positive, live a life you love. You can do this at any time: reset your habits, your diet, your sleep cycle, your relationships, your everything. It is always you; everything is you; how you decide to see things determines how you feel about things. You always have the power, the opportunity to change or see things differently.

Never give that power away to anyone thinking you are not in control. You are always in control of you and the inner you, the real you. You are always in control of your life and the way you decide to see others. You are entirely up to you; remember that. Release resistance.

Everything is possible. Open up to the possibilities. Work together with others. Your dreams can come true; many of them already have.

Remembering who you truly are, in a world that is constantly telling you who to be, what to do, how to think and how to live your life is the first step in taking back your power. We are constantly bombarded with rules and regulations, what's right and what's wrong, how to act in society, what to wear, how to be and so on. This can all get so confusing, and we can go off in search of good advice for this or that, only to receive so much that in the end we're still confused, still asking questions, and still feeling lost.

It is in the remembering, the recollection of who we truly are that revives that true sense of self. It allows you to live with confidence knowing you are listening and operating from the best source of information you can get, your true self guidance and all the wisdom and knowledge you hold inside. So, who are you? Do you even know the answer to that question? I am still on a journey of finding that out, or should I say remembering, but all I really need to remember is that inner voice and I know who I am, not my identity the world would like to give me but the real me. I believe we all come into this world with our soul's identity, our blueprint if you like, and then slowly over time like a jumper that's been through the wash over and over and forms bobbles of lint, we pick up parts of what becomes 'us' along the way. We also get a lot of labels. It starts when we're young, oh she's the sporty one, he's the academic one and she's the arty one, along with our physical looks, hair type, or eye colour. Then it might branch out into the rich one, the one with that car or that boyfriend or those amazing children who live in this place and travel there every so often and own this or that etc., etc. It's true that these things may form part of our new identity, our habits and so on but it is not our unique self, the real us, for the real us is not so concerned with our material world. The real self is concerned with shining its own brilliant light and not for the sake of showing off, as that would be the human ego, but to shine a brilliant light for others, on others and looking to unite with others' light.

I would say if you've truly found yourself, you've found yourself somewhere there, somewhere strange and in between but feels like home to you. Somewhere not exactly the same as 'anyone' else, not even your close friends and confidants.

In finding yourself you will also find a confidence, not like the confidence you feel when a pair of jeans fits just right and enhances some of your best assets, but a solid, internal, wind can't just blow over, kind of confidence. You benefit most from drawing on your inner light, strength, and soul that you have found inside of you. You don't feel the 'need' to be a part of any group, following or parade and in fact you are very careful and selective about who and what becomes an influence from the outside in. I say the outside in as I think about the individual in layers, in that we can allow our soul to radiate from the inside outwards and take up space in the world being exactly who we are, or we can be radiated on from the outside in, until it fills up all the space within us and we no longer remember or know who we are.

Personal Power

Spending some time with yourself and creating the space, and taking your personal power and vitality back have to be some of the most important things you can do for yourself in this fast-paced world.

Just when you thought you needed something, life was dull, you longed for something or someone, a new land perhaps, in those moments you take for yourself as personal time you will find yourself. You'll find yourself in that moment when no one else is around and it can be far from lonely. It can be more expansive than ever and in fact somehow in some way after connecting with your brilliant self you can begin to connect with others on an energetic level like no other. Your heart may begin to expand out to those you resonate with and they don't even have to be there physically for you to feel a connection.

You can revive and so can your world around you, but when did it feel like your soul self disappeared? It most likely disappeared a thousand times you didn't make time for yourself, time to spend with that person that has always been and will always be your constant. I'm referring to your amazing spirit, the one you see in the eyes of every child on this planet because they are still so connected to themselves and also the ones you see in the aged nearer the end of their life, who are now closest to the spirit world once again.

After all is said and done, when you open up so does your life! Sometimes it's so hard to get there when you're taking care of everyone and everything else. I thought that would stop when my children finally went off to school. Oh no, it never stops so you have to make some time for yourself, create the space, create your world.

It won't come to you by waiting or even by meditating. So go out into the wild, into the woods, or into yourself, whatever it is you need and remember that beautiful you.

This is called taking back your power, taking back your vitality, claiming your life like you claim each breath you inhale and sometimes all you have to do is start spending some time alone to get connected again. Connect with yourself and then connect with what vibrates with your world. It's important to find what you love, find what you resonate with. It could be an incredible song or soundtrack, singing, dancing, walking in nature, cooking or creating something.

It might be finding joy or love in animals or your favourite sport or activity, but it needs to be something you can find yourself in through reflection, something that mirrors your beautiful soul or you can 'feel' yourself through. It could be the power you feel in your body when you conquer that fitness class, the vitality that comes right up from your belly, where your power lies after eating a wholesome meal you just created or the feeling of excitement you get when a new idea breathes that zest for life within you or you become proud of yourself after completing something meaningful to you. Your personal power.

Inner Strength

Recently I stumbled upon a photo of me as a young child about 7 or 8 years old. I was carrying the family's backpack for the day as we were on a trek somewhere. The backpack looked fully loaded and I've realised as an adult that I was probably trying to prove my strength to my family by carrying it. It occurred to me even then the conditioning we take on as young children to try to be seen, be heard, validated and loved. That physical masculine strength was somehow praised over any inner strength of being who you truly are, perhaps soft, gentle, or feminine.

What hurts and saddens me the most about growing up in our western society of money, dominance and competition is the lost souls that still lie dormant within.

The many years throughout my childhood I thought I somehow had to prove myself with outer strength. I did this through cross country running in primary and secondary school, but for the most part I didn't actually enjoy running. With the familiar burn in my chest, lower back pain, and ache in my legs, I pushed through. I enjoyed winning but mostly I enjoyed praise, and I enjoyed being someone that did something that was recognised in this world as important or an achievement.

The same could be said for being the top of the class in mathematics in primary school; like a monkey I would perform. How trainable we are when we are afraid of showing our true selves, when we conform to the praises of the world and what other people deem an achievement. These days an achievement to me, is being my true self out in public and paving my own way in life. That to me is true strength.

So, all along my true strength lay within. I knew this of course on some level even as a child, but kept it hidden like a treasure in a box, perhaps thinking it was meant for some other land in another time. I see now that it is this world that needed my inner strength, needed me to show the world on the outside what was on the inside, and that all my softness, qualities and gifts that come from a pure heart are what this world is so in dire need of. Now that, I'd like to be a leader of, a leader of love, a leader of inner strength, a leader of being my true self, unafraid.

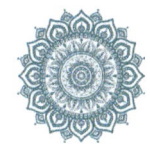

chapter 4
remember soul love

"If love is universal, no one can be left out."
DEEPAK CHOPRA

A Deep Hearted Connection

As much as there is so much help out there, so many resources, so much selfhelp material, we all still need so much help! We're not done yet; we're still searching, still healing, and some of us have not even begun or don't know where to begin.

Perhaps it is more about what's on the inside than on the outside. Perhaps it is in the stillness, the quiet and the reflection that we remember what we are deeply connected to or not. For a deep-hearted connection, we must go deep and allow whatever is there to come to the surface. If it is too hard to sit with what might be coming up for you, maybe you need to scream, maybe you need to cry, stretch it out, write, dance, swim it out or run. Move the energy. Whatever comes naturally or feels normal to you, do that; it doesn't matter what other people think; you are doing you.

Not once have I ever witnessed in all the many yoga classes I've ever taught anyone being angry at each other at the end of it. Yet we were all very, very, different: different body types, face shapes, skin colouring, abilities, jobs, points of views, religions, etc. Not once was there ever apparent conflict amongst two people. I taught a lot about nonjudgement; it was almost my favourite part of yogic philosophy.

You see, it's not that we weren't being ourselves at the end of each yoga class; on the contrary, we were closer to our true selves more than ever after we'd tuned in, dropped our judging human ego minds and opened up our hearts.

We loved ourselves unconditionally at that point and we respected each other. Strive to stay in the love as much as you can for a life lived from your pure essence, your soul self.

If you're ever looking to feel or experience expansion, try opening your heart. There are many ways in which to do this. You can picture your heart chakra like a lotus that closes at night and opens wide to receive the sun's rays by day.

When it's open wide it is the most beautiful and the most radiant. When it is closed it sits in deep reflection under the moon shine. Both ways in which it finds itself have purpose and are required for the health of the lotus; however, you will rarely see it unopened in the day when the sun is shining.

As humans we can close off our heart chakra when we feel the cold or the dark penetrate us from external or internal sources. It could be from our own thoughts or thoughts of others. With us too there is a time to close and a time to open; however, sometimes we can forget to open, especially if an event has been traumatic for our sensitive hearts. It's time to remember your soul love that you have inside.

Making the Connection

Life has always had a way of jolting me back to reality, reminding me sometimes harshly with a thud, like falling back to Earth, that I am here to connect with others in this present time, and perhaps my job is to bring messages. I am coming to understand that that is my duty, no, my service that I can offer to the world. I am in flow when I am writing, when I am downloading, and this is my true happy place.

My point is this: if there were no others in this world to connect with, how could I know myself? In my instance, who would I write for? With whom would we share our gifts? You see other people help us in knowing ourselves better.

We get feedback from them that teaches us about who we are and even more so, we learn about who we are by giving feedback to others. We learn what we have inside of us and what we are capable of. What would

I have to reflect upon? How would I see my shadow or look in the mirror if it wasn't for other people? Sure, I could always look to nature (the sun reflects off the moon; the lake gives us a reflection) but we are afforded a whole tapestry of learning through our relationships and interactions with others.

It's so important to know and embody your gifts, but it's also important to be able to make that heart and soul connection with others so you can share your soul self with the world to really make a difference.

A Lens Through the Eye of the Storm

If we could operate on a soul level at all times, I wouldn't ever have needed to write this book; however, we are in fact souls having a human experience and a human experience we shall have. We come hardwired with a myriad of emotions right from birth. We mostly come into this world as pure love and light, perhaps minus some past life karmic baggage that we have to work off in this lifetime.

In the first seven years of our life we begin to be conditioned and programmed and our network of emotions begin to associate with different experiences contributing to the way we think about ourselves and the world around us. Our minds often get busier and louder and even go on autopilot and our inner voice or true self as we go out into the world gets quieter. So, unless we literally connect in and resonate and revive our souls each day we go along and tend to forget who we really are amidst the noise and haste.

Meditation is one of the simplest, most accessible forms of getting close to who you truly are; it is your lens through the eye of the storm. It is a way to get in touch with your higher self, quieten the noise around you, and remember the soul within and the love that is you.

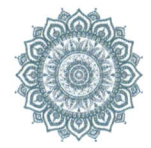

chapter 5
remember soul speak

"Don't shush your inner voice; it's who you really are."

AUTHOR UNKNOWN

The Expression of Your Soul

We come in knowing who we are and what we want; we just have to reconnect to remember. How often do we truly feel our being emanate through us? In the quiet times certainly, and as I write this book for sure. But how and when else are we truly being who we truly are? We are human most of the time as our lives are jam-packed and too busy to be listening to our soul speak on the inside.

There can be so many distractions and disturbances throughout our day even when we try and take a moment's peace, whether it is work, caring for children or someone else, and just all the responsibilities of the day to day. A daily moment's peace is imperative even if it's a 10-minute cuppa in silence, a moment to gather our thoughts and then let them go, to come back home to our true self.

I had a hand analysis done a few years ago (different from palm reading), and it showed that I was from the school of peace and love. It's no wonder I am a peace seeker or is it really that I'm seeking what's within that peace? Perhaps I'm seeking a space to find myself in any given moment, to hear my own thoughts, to hear my soul speak. No wonder writing feels like an indulgence to me, a space to hear my soul speak, where thoughts flow and words are released onto the page. What an outlet!

If I'm honest it's when I'm my best self more often, when I'm getting time to myself to reflect, meditate and be in creative flow. I'm a happier person because my soul is so happy that it gets to come alive and shine through on the pages, that it gets to bring out the expression of itself. Literally, it gets to live! I can only hope my words bring comfort or inspiration to my readers as much as they do to me. You are truly your own best friend, lover and confidant, the person you've always been searching for. Everything we crave or desire is within us. We look outside desiring everything that is already within; it is just waiting to be noticed and expressed on the outside.

How can we know what we want if we don't know who we are? I recently completed a vision board and allowed the drive of what my soul really wants to experience in this life to come through. It turns out there are about three things on my board that I'm currently working on or have already dabbled in and the rest are new experiences yet to come. It can be an interesting exercise to do as I notice most of what I really want is not currently in my life. That's okay; I have time and most importantly a vision for it that I can slowly call into my life. It is not made up of shiny cars, diamond rings, and houses, but of places, experiences, new knowledge, and activities. There is nothing wrong with cars, diamonds, or houses either, but I know my soul is speaking to me when it becomes about experiences it wants to have versus material items.

Material items can also be an experience that the soul may desire so there is nothing wrong with that; it's just my soul at this time does not want for that. I know this because I know what I truly want on a soul level because I spend the time to get to know the real me amongst the chaos of life. When I know what I want on a soul level I feel fulfilled when I achieve this.

Recently I've had this picture of me on my bedside table of when I was about 7 years old. I've been connecting into the photo and through it, to that inner child that still lives within me. That child at the time would have been so much closer more often to her soul self. Only being in the world for such a short amount of time she was a true reflection before she was influenced by the world around her through her experiences and what she learnt. It was before her ego sought to protect her fiercely from any fear or past experiences and before she learnt to wear a mask and present to the world the way she had learned the world wanted her to be. So pure and born with inner wisdom from past lives and experiences she was her soul self, but with memory or connection on a conscious level to this erased. My soul self is gentle, sensitive, wise, and caring of others. She is love and peace but also adventure. She is intelligent and, in this body, physically strong and healthy, fast when she needs to be. Along the way I remembered my fire within.

Our soul incarnates and adapts to the world around us; like waves crashing into rock, we are moulded and shaped to our environment. We pick up on the behaviours of the people around us and they become our influences. Thus, the expression of our souls, unless given the opportunity to be drawn out, is somewhat supressed without us even realising.

It's time to remember you. You could try a photo meditation if you can find one of you when you were a young child. Find a quiet space and really study the photo. Look at the expression on your face. What were you doing, feeling at the time? It can help to connect with who you truly are, to jog your mind, heart, and most importantly, soul. It's been waiting for you all this time to remember.

Rejection as a Barrier to Your Truest Expression

Rejection, no place for the ego self. When we come more and more into our truth and we shake off the conditioning that has led us to feel shame or have judgement, we are acting as our authentic self. This means being our true self comes less from a place of courage and more from a grounded standpoint where the ego does not get involved and where we can speak our truth from a pure state. We need to be in quite a conscious state to ensure we are not acting from our ego self that will ultimately bring fear, hurt or rejection. Anytime we find ourselves rejecting our truth or others' truths, the ego is at work. It's time to check in and see where this wound is within us that needs healing. Whether we perceive something to be weakness, ugliness, less than expected, not up to standard, we have a deep wound to attend to.

We need to ask ourselves where this judgement is coming from and where our love and compassion has gone. Always coming back to your authentic self, the gentle soft whispers that you find in the essence of you will guide you. The ego is there to protect you; however, most of our egos in this modern world have run rampant as we fear rejection. The cycle continues and spins on until we say stop, until we say no more, until we become conscious.

Next time you wish to speak your truth and find fear rising in you from judgement, try nonjudgement on for size and stick to your soul's truth. Take courage from your spirit's whispers and know your spirit holds you steady and safe as you show up more and more in this world as your true self. Remember who you truly are and allow your soul to speak up.

The Rise and Fall

Today I fell hard. Everything just hurt all at once and my body was heavy and felt the pull of gravity. I surrendered to the pain and the chaos and the heartache and the numbness all at once. I let my anger and frustrations out and I let my tears rise from my throat and flow through my eyes, into my hands. I let mother Earth catch me and my husband's hand hold mine while my head found his knee to rest on. I was on the floor in a pile of emptiness whilst surrounded by mess.

Isn't it funny when we push and we fuss and we fight and we think we have it all together and the strength of our souls to hold us, and then all of life suddenly weighs us down and we don't?

When we surrender and fall to the floor, something magic happens to us. We find mother Earth holding us and we can fall no more. We find peace in a few hours of silence while our head empties and body replenishes. We find our hearts a little less broken and we realise it is this earthly realm that holds our soul after all. We remember we are human and may be broken sometimes but we always rise again. After we have surrender ourselves to the Earth, to our mortal selves, then we may reclaim who we truly are once again and rise slowly and steadily as we walk our path like a tightrope walker, cautiously one foot in front of the other.

Perhaps the realisation that comes after this journey, each time with the rise and fall, is how very human we are, yet heavenly all at once. We realize how there is always such a thin veil; one comes with a thud and the other with our feet lifting off the ground. Somewhere in between, our emotions are rattled, as if in the path of a hurricane, and then there is always the calm after our storm has blown over. Then we pick ourselves up, sometimes having to peel ourselves off the ground, and walk on.

chapter 6
remember soul sees

"You can remember it if you want by unravelling the double helix of inner knowing."

CHERIE CARTER - SCOTT

A Window to Your Soul Self

I've always felt so connected to my soul self. I always had that relationship right from the start, just never knew it. Chances are if you've read this book this far, you now realise you have too if not before. It wasn't until adulthood that I became aware that the sensitive part of me, the inner knowing, the subtle buzzing vibration or other alerting sensations going on inside me was actually my soul self.

Growing up I used to find it such an inconvenience as it seemed to be the signal to the things that triggered me and caused me pain in my life. I used to see it as something that bothered me versus realising it was something that was there to help me. It would let me know when things were not okay and when they were.

Not until adulthood, did I learn how to utilize this gift by discerning, interpreting and tapping into this intuition.

Some may relate to their intuition as the pleasure or pain feelings of an energetic nature. I take this type of pain as a sign to check in with my soul self to see what is going on and what direction I should go next. Yes, it is our inner guidance system that some may relate to as bodily intuition on an energy level, and really what that intuition is giving us is a window to our soul self. A message it is trying to tell us through subtle signs, gut instincts and inner wisdom.

The third eye in yogic philosophy is for us to take a deeper look on the inside as opposed to our two human eyes that are to look outside of ourselves. The third eye can be drawn or known to be reversed facing inwards for that very reason as that is its purpose. These vibrations that we can feel in our bellies or whole body usually lets us know that we need to make some adjustments in our external or internal environment and that our soul is not in alignment or agreement with what we have come across at any time in our lives.

When we are aware of our intuition and its purpose, we can become tuned in and use it as a personal navigation system for life. It pays to know about and remember this ancient part of ourselves, that again serves as a messenger from our soul in a vibrational way. It is a long last part of our intelligence that we have been steered away from in modern life and it is time to trust it once again. It is part of our personal power after all.

Trusting Your Innate Knowing

We all have our own internal navigation system that will never let us down.

The vibrations we feel, the things that trigger us, lead us to our true self. If we are triggered vibrationally it will run through our whole body or in our belly; that is our instinct saying something is off here or telling us to run! If we are triggered in our heart centre, there is a wound waiting to be healed and it is most likely a life lesson of ours to overcome. That kind of trigger we breathe through, investigate perhaps and do some more 'work' on so that we can overcome the lesson or facilitate the healing that might be needed .

The other kind that is a strong vibrational warning, that is your soul speaking to you, it is not one to ignore. This does not mean you need to run and hide, but trust the vibrations and act accordingly. Not to be dismissed, this is your inner navigation system. It is designed so that you can stay on the path of that which is your true self. When you follow your intuitive instincts, you won't ever have to worry whether you are going in the wrong direction in a situation or life itself.

You will be living in alignment with who you truly are and unfolding perfectly as you were meant to.

Unique Perceptions

The way you see yourself reflected in the mirror is nothing like others see you. From fine details to how your hair falls across your face and from the angle you see it will be very different to the angle others see, and that's just your physical appearance.

Perceptions, as I have come to understand, are as unique as your own fingerprint. In fact, the 7 billion plus people on the planet, if they were to all meet you, would each see you differently. Perhaps some would see you similarly, but none would see you exactly the same as another would. This is what your eyes see from their vantage point.

Remember that what your soul sees, is also from a unique perception and that we have the ability to tap into our higher self awareness and expand our vision of what we see. Unlike the human eye we can use the power of our intuition to gain new insights. Even the word insight, to me explains things we couldn't see before but when we look within and search from a higher self we are able to come up with a new vision we had not known before.

Until we awaken our higher self, develop the relationship using our third eye (inward looking sight) we remain with the use only of our human eyes. That's not to say that that is not a miracle in itself when we look at the world around us, but when we remember the power of who we truly are, we are given sight that is beyond our unique perceptions and something truly not of this world. The real power then, is when we are able to use our intuition for the benefit and good of all and the planet we live on. To help make the world a better place, to see danger where there is real danger and to discern when there is not. To feel the world through vibration and allow our sixth senses to guide us, live a magical and wonderful life to the fullest as we harness our true power within.

chapter 7
remember soul connect

"Awareness of the inner body is consciousness remembering its origin and returning to the source."

ECKHART TOLLE

Lightness of Your Soul

Most of my topics or themes come to me through my personal life experiences, reflections, musings, and no doubt my soul self. My soul self frequently drops me some pretty amazing insights and inspiration to work with and articulate into comprehendible material. My inner voice gets loud when my world gets quiet, and I tend to go with it, since it proves itself time and time again to be rather wise and positive.

I believe we all have this within us; we just need to get really quiet and hear our soul speak which has all our best interests at heart. You'll know when it's your soul speaking because it will flow. It won't question anything and will make sense of everything. It usually runs like a tap, is plentiful and literally could continue to run on autopilot if you let it.

It is important, however, to be grounded, and we need to come back into the present moment afterwards for the practicals and interactions of life. This is usually when it seems to shut off for me, anyhow. The world gets noisy and we begin to listen to others as we need to communicate and be fully present.

Just remember to connect with the lightness of your soul as often as you can for guidance and especially when the world feels heavy. Create a space for yourself; some may call it an altar. You might like to use candles or incense, play soft music, whatever speaks relaxation to you. It's important to set yourself an intention before you rest into meditation, focus on your breathing, or just allow your daily thoughts to float away for a time. The intention could be to connect to your soul self.

The more we spend time with our soul self though, the more we nurture it, the stronger it becomes, and we start to operate more from that space. When we tap in and connect with our soul self, we start to make important decisions from a calm, centred, rational and heart driven space instead of our conditioned subconscious mind that can often be fearful, irrational, pressured and worrisome. That is when we become aware of who we truly are and how freaking powerful and amazing our immortal self is. We get the feeling like our feet are lifting off the ground instead of dragging concrete around. It's a nice place to stay but remember we are here to be human first and foremost with our souls as our guiding light.

Awakening to What's Within

While we're all looking out there for direction, inspiration, and the answers to life, the fact is, it all lies within us. Our whole world spins and swirls inside of us waiting to be born on the outside, waiting until we are ready to look inside and bring it into this world of creation and materialise our dreams into reality. Sounds simple enough, right? Well, as we all know, there is this thing called life that happens on the outside of us that has been manifesting since before birth and before we became fully aware of our power to create our own reality.

While we were growing up, we were mostly unconscious of this power or the knowledge that we create our own reality with our thoughts and feelings and what we hold inside. We were under the illusion of thinking we had no power as a child and began to be programmed through our subconscious from the outside world. We were children and we mostly did as we were told even against our free will, out of fear of punishment, rejection, or pain. We are in survival mode from the moment we are born as we rely on the people around us for our basic needs. We then, however, began to rely on the people around us for our source of joy and so we continued to comply with the outside world.

At a child's level this might look like, "be a good boy or girl and you will be rewarded with lollies or toys" or sadly sometimes even affection and love was a reward in exchange for compliance. We often were led to believe power was outside of us and became our game called life. We had no idea of what our personal power was (more on that later in this book), let alone dared to speak it for ridicule or judgement if in fact we even knew what our own truth was.

Finally, we began to trust in others more than our own innate wisdom, intuition, and knowledge. We left ourselves behind and forgot the place we came from before landing on this planet, the grand universe, and we forgot we are as grand as the universe too. Nobody thought to tell us because chances are our own parents and their parents and so on have gone through this same process too.

Even if they had glimpses of awakening to their own self throughout life, and life may bring hardship for this to happen, quite often they were not in a world that was supportive or conducive to the individual living life on their terms. Quite the opposite, in fact people are easier to control when they are either none the wiser of their power within or living in fear.

When we remember our soul self, we awaken to a power within like no other, one capable of leading us and guiding us through life with our highest interests at heart, our purpose in hand and the potential to create lasting positive changes and impacts here on Earth.

Remembering Our Connection

I think we've forgotten who we truly are, I really do. I'm not surprised and it's not our fault either. This goes back centuries and it's a long story.

For the most part, and in today's world, you're probably not surprised either.

When do we ever stop to take a breath? On our annual leave over four weeks a year maybe, but then not really, because then there are holiday pressures. There are the kids, play dates, entertainment, family and friend commitments, financials to contend with and so on.

We never stop. The world is spinning so fast and seemingly out of our control, so when do we ever get to grasp the side of this spinning wheel and get off?

We do when we decide to. When we say enough. When our soul screams at us, when it is time to awaken.

Awaken. What do we mean by that? It's a word that's used often, perhaps along with enlightenment. Here's my take in the context of this writing anyhow.

To awaken to me means, literally, to wake up for a moment or a series of moments from the dream or illusion that we are living day to day. Meaning, when we are racing around 'doing' what 'needs' to be done we are for the most part 'asleep' to ourselves and in automatic mode. We are not feeling particularly inspired, we are not allowing for our soul to be leading the way we are in human mode.

It's okay; we need that; we are human and that's fine but if we want to be living an inspired life or we have a driving force coming from our soul within it may pay to stop from time to time to allow for that to come through.

Easier said than done, I know; you will have to carve out some time, set some boundaries and put yourself first; it's imperative.

You will have to let those around you know what you're about and what you intend to do. Others do not have to believe in you and sadly most of your family and friends won't, except for the ones who may be trying to do the same thing, understand you or are on the same path.

When we awaken to who we truly are there is kind of no going back. It's a journey, one on a winding road and sometimes in reverse but there is no falling back asleep, perhaps only momentarily or on purpose sometimes as we try to run away from our true self.

Why would we want to run away from our true self? It's because our true self truly challenges us. Life is a challenge and that's why most of us came here so your true self is going to make sure, once you are aware, that you stay awake and stay true to your path.

I believe in flow, I really do, but I also believe with the life we have and the world we live in when we are 'not there yet' requires us to fight for our right to party. Meaning, we can know who we are, be as gifted as possible and still not be living the life our soul intended to.

It may take some grit and definitely some sacrifices. I don't really love the word hustle. After all, our soul is not here to fight through the crowd but to shine through the storms and keep rising.

chapter 8
remember soul search

"And all along my heart was searching for what my soul already knew."

ALEXA

Rainbow In a Dark Sky

So today I am not so okay. I mean, in reality, on the surface I'm okay but what's paddling beneath is not so good. There are ripples that won't settle; there is a mind full of life that's racing from topic to topic. I've tried music, yoga, grounding my feet on the earth, cooking and a good cup of tea. Whatever is in me today is not settling; perhaps it's not supposed to. It's like a clash of sensitive energy versus go, go, go, versus I don't want to go, and I feel exhausted emotionally.

Today is a designated day to write this book and I don't feel so shiny. I don't feel inspiring today. I am grateful to be able to write how I'm feeling. I feel lonely and I know that this is all normal too. I feel like my barrier to feeling better is trying to feel better. What if I stopped trying for a moment? What if I accepted it and accepted myself and loved myself in my feelings of blue anyhow? What if that was the key to feeling better? What if I am all I need? Just me, my allowance of space to feel and myself. Myself as my guide, my strength, my all.

What if I told you I'm already starting to breathe a little easier in this knowledge of allowing? What if this knowledge that provides comfort becomes the rainbow in my dark cloud today? What if that is all I need to catch me as I fall? Because how can we always be so shiny? Well, in truth we are not. Perhaps we are, in fact, equal parts light and equal parts dark.

How much in society do we push for a smile; a fake, light conversation; and grab that mask and put it on so tightly that we can't even begin to breathe? How much are we trained or taught to be okay? You know what, some days we are just not and that is perfectly okay. It is not all sunshine, lollipops, and rainbows, and I would like room in my life to not be okay without needing to explain it to anyone or even myself because perhaps like today I don't know why.

When did we stop allowing ourselves to go through and process life, to allow life to go through and process us? I am so grateful for my writing and for my book for they are as much my saviour as they might be yours reading through these pages. Today is a day

I get to be all by myself, and I've come crashing down so to speak. It's a day I become still with myself, one I usually seem to relish in and find lightness, energy and inspiration. Not today. Not today, but I am teaching myself that is perfectly okay. Today the 'inspirational' songs I usually play are not resonating; my body is tight and tired and sore and does not want to stretch much. My mind wants to fix everything, and my heart feels so heavy it feels like I can't even breathe. So, I will start from here today.

I will start from the very space I find myself in and I will stay there until it feels natural to shift into another mode. I honour the darkness in me as much as the light knowing how much more vibrant the colour of the rainbow looks against the colour of a dark cloud. Now that I have gotten that off my chest I can delve deeper now that I can breathe deeper.

The thing is, when we can accept our own darkness without feeling like we need to light it up we can accept everyone else's darkness in the world too. We learn to forgive; we learn where this darkness comes from; and we learn that dark clouds are just that, clouds, and they are temporary but do carry lessons and deep meaning. They carry signposts to follow and deep messages, and if we are willing to open the door and let them in like the hungry wolf at your door we have been taught to fear, we will see that the wolf carries messages of deep wisdom to share and messages of light.

soul self

Today I have come undone, and it is the best thing that could have happened to me. See, when you crack a little or a lot, all your pain gets to seep out, tears may flow, and you begin to feel like yourself again. You realise that perhaps you needed to break like the seed that splits before it grows into the plant that blooms. I begin to breathe; I begin to breathe deeply as I release and let go. We cannot always just release and let go; sometimes when we have built our shell so strong, we need to crack wide open to let the light in. We become so very undone, and we get to piece ourselves back together; it is all part of the process but we must allow it if we are to be led by the intelligence of our soul and trust our higher selves. Know that love is the way and that our souls want the best for us.

Anyhow, what a world it is that we live in. How could we just talk about the sunshine, lollipops, and rainbows but not talk about the struggles, the fear, and the pain we all go through? How negligent that would be. How untruthful and unauthentic that would be. Although I have left soul search to the end in each part, it is by no way the least important; it is part of the process we go through to get to the rainbow and a never-ending cycle. Each time it lifts us higher and higher on our journey of ascension as we heal and learn and grow. We grow through the darkness and the colours to reach the light.

I am so grateful for the darkness. I am even more grateful to be able to have the space, love, and acceptance for myself to allow myself to come undone, to give myself permission to not be okay when I am not and be the rainbow in my own dark sky. I hope you can too.

A little note. Have you seen the Japanese pots that have broken but get pieced back together with gold? They go from pots that look like every other pot to a beautiful most unique item that could never have been if it were not for it's journey in this life. Remember we search in the dark to find the light that will carry us forward. We are that light.

Glimpses of Soul Self

The challenge we face and the challenges we've always faced lie within our own abilities and commitments to the process of opening up and allowing the light to come in. It can be very daunting and very scary to face our own darkness or shadow self. The light being or spirit within us confirms to us our light and therefore it can bring contrast and be confusing to our human mind and ego that we could ever be anything other than love. We need to acknowledge the collective human consciousness that we are living through and that we as humans do, in fact, make mistakes and hurt one another.

This is not to say that each human that does wrong and has caused hurt should be condemned forever, no, quite the opposite. It is never our job to judge even when we are triggered to. We are not getting out of this collective human consciousness alone, so we need to find that forgiveness and compassion within ourselves, for ourselves, and for others no matter what. Hard to digest, hard to swallow I know when you think of the darkest acts against any human or living thing on our Earth. We must overcome this to free others so they may be allowed to heal, forgive themselves, and be brought into the light. As the quote from Martin Luther King Jr. states "Darkness never drives out darkness; only love can do that."

Nothing I've ever really read has ever really stuck with me for life except parts and fragments of certain theories, concepts or practices that have really resonated with my soul and therefore been easy to embody. So instead of looking on the outside for material to inspire and uplift we can simply just find it within ourselves in peace and silence and be certain to embody that. What you find inside is absolute gold because it is nothing short of absolutely what you need to live on the outside.

When we judge another, we are really judging ourselves. These glimpses of our soul self that we are afforded along our journey are a confirmation that no matter the darkness, we are the light.

Dark Days Bring New Awakenings

Recently I went through a heavy month of trauma. Trauma does not have to be something severe to be trauma; every pain you go through needs processing and healing. Never allow anyone to invalidate what is painful or traumatic for you, least of all yourself.

COVID-19 came to visit my family at the beginning of December. I fell sick first and then five or six days later, my husband, followed by my eldest daughter.

Our youngest never contracted it and my son contracted it when I was on day 14 and seemingly fully recovered. We spent Christmas in quarantine and had a very quiet New Year's.

COVID-19 itself for us was no more than a moderate virus in itself; however, its ability to highlight any underlying health conditions seemed to be its main focus. My asthma that had not been a problem since I was 14 flared up as did inflammation and hormonal issues. My husband and son were the same with health issues cropping up. This left us battling some health issues that we were not expecting for Christmas and into the new year. Of course, it was all a blessing in disguise as it made us pay serious attention to our health and set us on a path to become even stronger.

It did, however, place great strain on our family for a period there, with us all managing different health issues at once.

My point is that for a good six weeks my life was suddenly taken over with health concerns without any warning. Stress was a natural part of this process and at times fear also tried to creep in. With what we had to deal with within the family on a mental, emotional, spiritual, and physical level, it left us all a bit weary to say the least. Sometimes in life, you just cannot be prepared for what's around the corner, but I think that it's is all part of growing. If you were able to be fully prepared and sail through the ups and downs you wouldn't be growing or evolving. Was it the worst thing I've ever dealt with in my life? No; however, it was still stressful and hard as we grew through what we went through individually and collectively as a family. I'm pleased to say we were all in better positions a month later, but still getting there at the same time. Plans go on the back burner, both work and social, and it becomes a very hard time and a period of healing from the experience and of course on a deeper soul level.

Heal we do, grow we do, get stronger and wiser we do. It's all part of life and evolution. One of my favourite sayings I came up with for difficult times is we 'grow through what we go through'. We refine, get clearer, cleaner, leaner in a sense of letting go of what no longer serves us in our life anymore. I am always grateful for all my experiences (maybe not at the time with the hard ones) as they help evolve my soul and make up who I am today. It's unfortunately the part of life that we have to accept but it's the part that makes us human. It reminds us that we are here as our brilliant souls but going through the human experience no doubt. I believe we came here to teach and learn and grow. Our soul has put its hand up to have this human experience no matter what its purpose is on Earth. It's not always easy, but in the end it's always worth it.

We also have a bunch of choices to make, and I don't believe there is ever a right or wrong choice, just the consequences of the choices we make. I don't believe in good or bad, just evolution. We are all evolving at different paces which is why I think we evolve collectively; it is cleverly designed this way so that we can teach and learn from each other.

Where we are headed is the bigger question; however, I believe life across the universe and all dimensions is endless. It certainly puts things into perspective for me when I think bigger this way, that this life is such a short time in the life of our soul's journey. I believe we are here for such a short period in contrast to our soul's journey that it is likened to a short movie or series even.

It allows me to let go more, feel free, fearless, and courageous in this life. For such a short time we are here why would we not expand into life as much as possible? Let go of the shackles on our feet, mostly placed by society, the perceived fears, rules, or expectations. Come back to the soul and realise you are but taking a picture in this life.

What do you want your picture to look like when you look back and reflect on your life and story that was you? What do you want to see? How would you have wanted to grow? What do you want to leave as a lasting imprint as your time in this life on this planet? What's really important to you?

Difficult times can be hard, but they can also be refreshing. Like a snake that loses its skin, you shed and become a new and improved version of yourself. In essence, you become that future self you've been dreaming about and life goes on. We are here to love, to bring joy and peace and ease suffering in any which way we know how. We are here to be these miraculous things called humans whilst witnessing the journey through the eyes of our soul and playing our part in the greater collective evolution.

part 2
embody

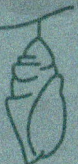

To Truly Love Who You Are Is to Truly Embody Your Soul Self

What does it mean to embody?

1. *Be an expression of or give a tangible or visible form to (an idea, quality, or feeling) – Oxford Dictionary*

To embody who you are is to bring the authentic you into existence, to feel into the authentic you, strip away what is not you or yours to carry and recognise what and who in fact that is. It's to give expression to, bring to life and show up as your original self. This part of the book is all about ways in which to begin to assimilate with the being within, to bring forward the life that has desired to be here and shine on every level. It's more than just an expression of you, but a definite tangible form and making the seemingly invisible part of you become visible, the part that is not just an idea, qualities or a feeling but the true self that lies within.

chapter 9
embody soul deep

"We are here to embody higher values and bring them into our world."

AUTHOR UNKNOWN

Embodiment Tools

Messages from your physical body..

Physical ailments are a sign that we need to bring attention to that part of the body, not so much for its physical sake but because there will be a deeper meaning and a deeper message surrounding it.

For example, once I was at a feminine embodiment and speaker training weekend that I'd been invited to by my sister-in-law. I had offered to help the hosts in exchange for being able to participate in the program. Working behind the scenes with people I had never met, doing tasks I had never done, was a very different experience to being a guest participant. I did not resonate with one of the hosts. Our personalities clashed. I found the person harsh and lacking the very feminine energy that was being promoted at the event. At the time, I felt I was in a position where I could not speak up as I had been 'lucky enough' supposedly to attend with an exchange of work, not money. I left the three-day event after 24 hours due to a sore throat that was quickly turning into tonsillitis.

The body can be very clever in getting your soul out of a situation it doesn't want to be in, if you are not speaking up and not feeling in alignment with what you are faced with. I was, perhaps, not rising to the personal challenge so to speak, not being my true self.

I wonder if I had spoken up about how I truly felt, given a voice to the soul part of me that felt supressed at the time, whether the sore throat would have eventuated. Experience has told me, time and time again, that perhaps it may not have come to that, that the sore throat was my soul pushing through to the body part of me. It was trying to let me know that whatever I was encountering was not resonating with my true self. My soul was not okay with what was going on and the lack of my expression about it. The irony was that it was a speaker training event. Clearly, I had some more work to do to gain courage, assertiveness, self-esteem perhaps and an honouring of my soul's true self.

Nonetheless, these life lessons come to us to help us stay true to ourselves and keep us on our path, the path that couldn't be more important, the honouring of our true selves and the living of a life in accordance with this.

If I'm honest, this was not an unfamiliar scene in my life experience so far.

Many times, in workplaces or social situations, I had felt like I could not speak up when I wanted to. It all comes back to wearing that mask and people pleasing no doubt and wanting to fit in or not cause a rift. These days I am living for me, what feels right for me and an honouring of my soul.

In most cases you will end up discovering that when you are not living for you, you are not really helping the people around you live for themselves either.

Being a shining example of living according to your soul's purpose and desire may cause rifts for some people but aren't we here to ruffle some feathers sometimes?

Aren't we here to cause a rift in a stiff world where not honouring your soul but doing things to be polite for the sake of others has been the norm? 'Do no harm' must firstly apply to yourself before you can preach it to others.

Have you ever felt that way, like you just couldn't speak up? What was the result of that for you? What do you think you need to be able to speak up in the future? Is it a deep self-love or needing to give yourself permission?

Our physical bodies are always giving us hints on where we might need to come more into alignment with our soul self. One of my favourite resources on physical ailments and what that might mean on a deeper level is from the late Louise Hay. 'You Can Heal Your Life' is a great publication of hers to give you some guidance on what our bodies (souls really) are trying to tell us. I believe when we are not in alignment with our soul self, in a place, relationship or situation, it shows up in our bodies.

Intuition – A deep connection to your soul self..

As long as I can remember, my soul has given me messages of guidance through many forms. One of the main ways has been through the body by way of physical ailments and physical sensations coming from intuitive signals.

Often these are signs we try to push away as they can make us feel uncomfortable at times. It could be sensations of butterflies in the belly, the heart pounding, the throat tightening, or an intense fear of a seemingly apparent threat, when we are in the presence of a person or place our soul is trying to tell us is not in the best alignment for us. If we dismiss these physical signals, it may not be in our best interests; we may end up in a situation that is undesirable or brings us to harm.

A story comes to mind of when my intuition (soul's signals) was strong and helped me out of a situation that could have been potentially threatening. I was down at the beach one day with my family and needed to go use the public toilets. There were stairs leading down to the toilets and the ladies' toilets were on the right. As I walked down the stairs, I noticed a man standing halfway down the stairs facing the toilets.

As I passed him my intuition leaped right out at me to be cautious of this man.

The sensations running through my body instantly put me into fight or flight stage and on alert. I had a strong feeling I would be followed into the toilets, but it was too late; I was already in. What unfolded next I believe was nothing short of my soul letting his soul know I was not only alert and aware to the fact that he may have been a threat, but I was ready to defend myself.

As I left my cubicle, I was ready for whatever came my way. I was in fight mode. I decided I would face this perpetrator head on; there was no other option. I had no phone with me, no way of calling for help. There was no one else around. I was it.

I expected that this person would walk into the ladies' toilets and follow me. I was right. I charged out of the cubicle. He was entering through the main toilet door. I stared him right in the eyes, let him know with all my soul that I was ready to defend myself if I needed to. I must have shocked him; he was not expecting that kind of a charge. I left quickly as I think he was left disillusioned.

It was set that I was not going to be a victim of anything. I was prewarned as my soul had leapt out at me and therefore ready for what was about to be thrown my way.

This state of alertness, allowing your conscious soul to lead the way in warning you sometimes of potential danger, is also part of embodying your soul self. It's letting your soul self come to the surface to be your keeper, your watcher, your alert system. That is not to say we need to live on high alert all the time, but just to be aware when we are getting the signs and signals from that intuition which is really our soul self alerting us. When the human part of us gets busy in life, caught up in life's dramas, stress or worries, we can fall unconscious and miss the beat sometimes instead of being in rhythm, in alignment with the soul voice within.

Yoga, meditation and accessing soul self-consciousness..

Through yoga practices and meditation, I have deepened my awareness of my soul's self-consciousness. I have learned mainly that the voice in my head, the mental chatter, is not my true self but mostly programming and noise on repeat.

I have learnt to develop a relationship with my soul self and learnt that it speaks to me from a different place. To be able to distinguish between our mental chatter and soul self means we can work to embody our soul self more often.

Our minds can then do the job of articulating what our soul wants to say; our hearts are there for the soul to experience emotions and our gut instincts are our soul speaking also. The vibrations we might feel, or an alignment or misalignment, is our soul calling out to us. There are many subtle bodies that our soul is connected to or connected through. The trick is to distinguish what is what so you can get closer to your pure self or consciousness, to be lead on a journey inwards, embody and journey outwards. Yoga or any meditation can be a practice to increase your awareness of the different parts of you: what is soul, what is human, and working together to become one, to become that highest human version of you possible in this lifetime.

The Chakras – Pranic/Energy Healing..

The seven main chakras are said to be energy centres of the body that pertain to different parts of the physical body and are associated with personal attributes, spiritual/life growth areas, and so much more. On our soul's journey this can be so relevant and provides us with guidance when it comes to being in alignment along our soul growth path.

There are many different methods, modes, and modalities that can assist you with finding out who you are which can help with embodying your soul self:

things that are personal to you, from your astrological birth chart from the time you were born to numerology which considers your birth date and its relevance to your soul's journey. There are Angel or Tarot cards that can be utilised to work with your higher self and the support of the universe, to crystals that can harness the kind of energy you need in any moment specific to you. Nutrition and naturopathy are relevant to the kind of food and herbs your body needs for optimum physical health; however, there are clues in here as to what your soul really needs, aligns to and resonates with for its purpose on this journey.

Following are some of the things I have used to know more about me, inside and out, to know more about the history of my soul and its purpose and to help me on my path. There really is no limit to what is available; this is just a short list that you might like to start with as you explore things for yourself.

Astrology, numerology, angel or tarot cards, healing crystals, essential oils, nutritional medicine, naturopath, massage, body spin, hand analysis, star seeds, yoga, yogic philosophy, pranic healing, meditation, personal development.

Who Am I?

People may often ponder, "Who am I?" Who are we in fact?

In our physical DNA, it is said that we are made up mostly of the seven generations who came before us, and we will also influence the next seven generations who come after us. This is also true of our mental, emotional, physical, and spiritual self as we influence the next generations and have been influenced by the past.

At our core being, our unique point of consciousness, the pure self if you like, we are but a vibrational match (or were at the time of birth) to the family and the geographic location we were born into on this Earth.

As we go along in life both of those things can and for the most part do change as we evolve one way or another. This, I believe, is part of our great purpose and is how we evolve and grow. Like a seed, we are not planted to remain a seed but to grow, bloom and transform.

Who you are today at this point as you read this book is a manifestation of the many layers and the life you have led and all of your experiences and influences up until this point. Like a magnet, you collect particles through your daily life, through the people and the places that surround you, through 'life' itself. For the most part, we often go around being nothing compared to who we truly are.

Unless we're getting quiet every day, switching off the noise around us and the thinking of our monkey minds, we're not really able to 'listen' or 'feel' our soul speak, so how could we possibly operate from there throughout our day? As part of embodying your soul self it's important to not only know who you are but to stay connected through regular reflection, moments of peace and quiet and awareness of the inner voice versus the mind's chatter also known as the monkey mind. We will do a better job of embodying our true selves when it becomes a habit, something that becomes a part of our everyday routine. Do you have a meditation practice or another embodiment tool that you use to harness your soul self everyday?

'When we get quiet, we get curious and when we get curious, great discoveries about who we are can be made and embodied.'

Who are we now then at our core? We are still a vibration that emanates quietly as we once did before we were given life in the human form, but we now carry layers of our life around with us. This might be a positive thing, this might be a negative thing and most likely a mix of both, but how do we get back in touch with our sacred vibration, our true being, consciousness that is our own?

The answer is in silence. Through silence – the silence that allows our soul to speak - and meditation techniques we can get really close and intimate with that core being. This doesn't mean you will hear your soul speak (although some people do); you might just feel it. I tend to feel my soul speak as it resonates within me. It is a calm, gentle, subtle, soft but powerful, immortal, and strong being, aged, wise and curious I am understanding. The more you get quiet, the louder or stronger you will hear or feel your natural self. You may have visions, insights, even smells and tastes, that come to you that feel like 'home'. Home that is not any particular home but a home within yourself, one that you just 'know' innately is who you truly are and it feels good.

A meditation practice that allows you to connect with your soul self on a deep level is a great way to embody who you truly are at your core.

What Is a Soul?

Light consciousness, consciousness, energy consciousness. What do we mean by consciousness? The observer, the witness, intelligence of some kind. For the lion to truly know its existence it must have a reflection; it may see itself in the water hole as it leans in to drink for the first time and it becomes aware of its physical existence or reflection, but who is noticing? The lion, of course, but what part of the lion? Is it the mind or the soul? The heart may fall in love with the sight or reflection, the mind may wonder or marvel at what it has seen, but it is the soul or the observer within the lion that becomes enlightened with new knowledge of itself, new intelligence, new consciousness that has expanded into new knowingness. It is the soul even after the lion's body has passed from its lifetime that will take its expanded consciousness in light source wherever its energy transfers or transforms to.

How do we know any of this for sure? It is my belief that all will be revealed as we pass this life and back into light consciousness held by source, God, the universe, or whatever you deem true for you. However, there have been people on Earth who have had near death experiences and recount what happened to them or what was on the other side. There are many, many reports also of children under 5 years old, able to tell adults exactly where they used to live and who they were in a past life.

There are also many other modalities that can tap into other realms, dimensions, and lifetimes to verify we are not just a human body having a human experience with a human heart and mind. I dare say if we were just flesh and blood, we may not even be able to have emotions, let alone the intuitive intelligence quite a few of us are able to tap into. There is definitely more at play; we are more than we could ever imagine, and the exciting thing is the more you remember your soul self the more you are able to embody all dimensions you are connected to, how great your soul is, and how very powerful you are able to be when it comes to shining your beautiful soul print on the world.

"The more we shine our light fully, the more we can be seen and potentially cause a flutter in someone else's darkness."

Healing, you see, has to happen first and then strength comes with awareness until you can be all of your true self all of the time and live exactly how you intended to before you came to this Earth.

Healing must be met at a person's current frequency and so if you have been drawn to this book enough to purchase it or found it came to you as a gift or in any other way, trust it is perfect for you at this time on your journey. It is my hope that you will be inspired to live a life as your true self, showing your true colours.

What could be worse than not living your life as your true self? Living your life according to other people's ideas, beliefs, values, or judgements. You are not here to be anyone else but you. Deep down, I know we are all pure spirit at our core; it is the layers that shadow our true selves. It is the fears, judgements, expectations, negative experiences, trauma and even our own ego that keeps us locked up in pain and living a life that is truly not our own. I am here to set me free and hopefully inspire you to do the same. Set your soul on fire? No thanks; I prefer to set my soul free, free from the inside out allowing my true self to emerge in all its glory.

"You are not required to set your soul on fire to keep other people warm." - Unknown

We are human beings, that means not just human but beings as well. Let's not keep our beings in the dark any longer and bring them to the surface. Let our beings live the inspired, aware, magic lives we were meant to live. We did not come to this planet to live small. Yes, you can take up space and paint a beautiful world for yourself.

My soul screams to share my thoughts, ideas, innate wisdom, and life lessons so I let it be and I let it be free. It is as much a gift to me first and will hopefully bring you joy, peace, understanding, comfort, knowing, freedom, awareness, insight and confidence to be the natural you.

It is my mission to inspire others to be exactly who they are on the inside on the outside as I travel that journey myself.

I believe if we could all feel accepted enough to be our true selves, take off the mask, we would achieve world peace. There would be no pretence, no rules, and no pain. I believe when there is no pain, there will be no suffering and we can all live as one.

What are your true colours exactly and how do you embody them? We are all born with our own set of unique soul level traits. This makes up who we are authentically. When we incarnate into a human body on this earthly plane, we also take on an ego. This ego serves to protect us but can also take on personas and influences of its own that don't reflect our pure spirit self. It can be tricky to navigate this life as our authentic self when we feel we've had to mask up or front up with an enlarged ego to fit in or protect ourselves from perceived harm (usually by the way of judgements from others). I hope this book encourages breaking down stereotypes, getting down deep into who you truly are and giving you the courage to not only feel truly comfortable and alive in your own skin but enable you to be brave enough to live a life you truly love and shine and inspire the world to do the same.

chapter 10
embody soul joy

"I've got joy like a fountain in my soul."
AUTHOR UNKNOWN

Learning From the Children of the World

Children just be themselves unapologetically and it's amazing! My three inspire me every single day. They have so much to teach us if we just stop, look, and listen. Whilst we as adults may find our children's behaviour challenging at times, I believe it is only because we have forgotten to allow ourselves to be ourselves and have been listening solely to our parents, teachers, influencers, and society for way too long.

At our core there is no naughty child or wrong doer; there is just the yearning to be who we truly are, and it is the same for our kids. We didn't come here to hurt anybody or cause trouble but to be our natural selves. 'Behaviour' happens when the soul is being squashed or suppressed in some way. Our children teach us to follow our instinctive heart's desire, live joyously, freely, and carefree. They do not, for the most part, carry the weight of the world on their shoulders from moment to moment.

Stopping and observing how children naturally honour the desire for joy within by pursuing it no matter what is going on around them, as if that's what they were born solely to do, is an inspiring way to remind yourself to do the same.

Taking a leaf out of their book is a great way to embody soul joy. As we go along in life, we can forget the things that matter most. We can forget that as much as we are here to grow, on the flip side we are here to glow. Life can get very serious, and we can get swept up in that, forgetting about our own joy within.

Feeling Our Own Joy Within

My boy of 16 was so concerned today that he doesn't have any friends and feels pretty down about what he is thinking about this situation for himself. He began a new school last year after we moved to a new area and then this year has seen school and sport club closures that has not helped with socialisation and creating new friendships. I know he has one or two good friendships going but perhaps not enough to fill his social desires. This can be a true heart breaker for a parent to hear from his or her child; however, I proceeded to ask him if he could just let this go for a moment and hear me out.

I told him that the best friend he'll ever have is himself and that when we solely look on the outside to fill our joyful desires, we miss that amazing human on the inside. I know this because it's what I used to do before my own soul self-realisation before I remembered and experienced the light that is me. I went on to explain that whatever he thinks he is looking for on the outside for himself is already there within him, that he is the most incredible human being that he will ever meet hands down, ever.

We are the awesomeness that we are always seeking. Nothing else will lift him higher than his own spirit and knowing and feeling that spirit inside that is him. The knowledge, the wisdom, and the answers that he seeks are all there. We are born with all our light, and we don't ever lose it, but as we get older we need to uncover or remember it. We are capable and powerful enough to feel our own joy whenever we want to tap in.

We are here to give as much as we are here to seek. I reminded him he is sixteen, this is a tricky transitional time to young adulthood, everyone would feel what he is feeling, and all the love and support is around him but mostly within him. That said, this was a lesson to feel the joy of the amazing being within first. Friendships are an important part of our growth and joy in this life and we all seek connection, that is a healthy part of life. It's just as important to remember and be connected to ourselves too. That part of us that is our constant in life, always having our own back. Find strength and resilience from within.

Filling Your Own Cup First

Do what makes you happy. Put yourself first, and then you will be lovely and liberate others to do the same. You will shine like gold as you walk down the street and the sparkle in your eyes and smile may spark something in others.

Never underestimate the power of satisfying your own needs first; you are that powerful for it to set off a chain reaction. The destiny of the whole universe really can lie within you if you believe in it enough. The question is, will you be brave enough to consistently aim to be in the mode of love to set off that chain reaction with yourself first and then all others that you come across? Be that light; be that shining beacon?

When we fill up our own cup first, give to ourselves, attend to our own needs, it is not selfish, it is self care. We give permission and show others how to care for themselves. We embody the love that we truly are and we encourage other's to do the same. We take responsibility for ourselves, for our lives, for our personal healing. We become the light, love and joy to those around us. We become leaders in a more nourishing way of living, remembering who we truly are meant to be. Let our cup of self love and joy overflow and spill out onto the world.

chapter 11
embody soul will

"It is not your environment, it is you – the quality of your minds, the integrity of your souls, and the determination of your wills – that will decide your future and shape your lives."

BENJAMIN E. MAYS

Boundaries

Two nights ago as I lay in bed, right before I fell asleep, I told my husband I felt so unhappy as I reflected on my day-to-day life. Here I am happy with the time and lifestyle I've created for myself, my new business and opening up to other new pursuits, but something just didn't sit right. I dived into my truth and feelings and allowed it all to surface. Turns out I'm feeling robbed of my time when it comes to pursuing my purpose. There just always seems to be demands on my soul (which is happy to help) but an unhealthy balance has crept in and is stealing my mojo. Yes, it's partly a mummy thing but it is more than that. It is not personally pursuing my purpose for too long. It is allowing 'life' to have taken over and not prioritising my special self or giving me the love and energy that I so freely give out. It is from putting my soul in the back seat and letting others sit up front. Was it a relaxed, conscious decision to do so? Hell no. Every morning when I wake up there are going to be a thousand things that day that potentially could steal my time. There are a thousand things pulling and tugging at me to go in this direction or that direction. It's like a tsunami everyday gathering me up while I wave goodbye and all my dreams get washed away.

Yes, the struggle is real. Imagine if I don't stand up for myself and say well no, I'm sorry, I'm going in this direction instead. There are then potentially a thousand things of unimaginable greatness within me that I am not providing space for or setting free into this world. It is time to stand up and say no and make more conscious choices. It's time not to push or struggle along with this but to rise tall to life's demands and let it know who's boss and who's in charge of my life path. Not in an arrogant way, but in a certain way, that I am certain this is what I am next bringing into the world. Let my soul lead and my head and heart dance to her beat along the way. This is me raw and real.

Courage Is for Survival

"Courage fired up with bravery and that fuelling of fear, not of what is to be conquered, but what will

conquer you if you do not face what you must, is the adaptation that is sometimes needed for survival."

Conscious courage has a place in our world when it comes to survival, but not as we've been led to believe in society when it comes to speaking up or being our true self.

We have learnt to stay quiet or risk feeling shamed, judged, or rejected by our brothers and sisters who have learnt to judge, shame and reject (usually the status quo) because of what they have learnt along their journey to believe. We have even learnt to gang up, bully and pressure others' narratives, points of views, and opinions.

Depending on which country you live in, you may be silenced or even killed for speaking up or sharing your views. Sadly, this is currently even happening in my country (the silencing by authorities on opposing opinions to the government's narrative). Yes, in 2021, in Australia people are being arrested, jailed and silenced for speaking up as they share their opposing views. All this aside, I say conscious courage is a survival technique required when you are being threatened in some way and in situations where your freedom, basic human rights, livelihood, or life is being threatened.

Freedom of speech, however, in general in society, is generally not a threat in most western countries. Sometimes we see it as this way though, as suggested earlier when our brothers and sisters oppose what we are saying, so we stay silent. At least I did for a lot of my life and I am still learning to implement in my daily life what I believe is needed (and it's surprisingly not courage) to speak up.

What I believe is needed is firstly a deep connection to ourselves, a knowing of our true self. With this comes an attitude of non-judgement as we connect with our spirit and realise we are here to love, to serve, and to bring peace. Below the layers, we naturally have an awareness that is non-judgemental and is compassionate, understanding and forgiving. We realise the human suit we are wearing is mortal and for the time that we are here our job goes way beyond and above judging others. When we begin to operate from this soul level as we get in touch with it more often, we naturally become less judging, shaming, blaming and so on. We realise our brilliance, our light, our shine and we rise above such limiting situations and beliefs.

I remember one of my yoga teachers saying if you are feeling judged then teach non-judgement. Pretty soon it becomes your new narrative and when you are not judging other souls it is hard to feel judged or even judge yourself. For me and for most of us I bet, we are our biggest inner critics. I have also found the power of recognising your own brilliant gifts and talents and what you have to bring to the world coupled with a big dose of self-love and appreciation can be a great antidote to self-judgement. It is where our inspiration lies and what our self-worth and confidence is tied to.

Also, a very grounded and humbling point of view of the self is a sure way to keep you steady when you are speaking up in public or amongst friends and family. At the end of the day, courage has no place in a social setting unless your life is being threatened. Think about that next time when you feel fear, that your life is not being threatened, just your negative human thoughts or maybe someone else's which is their job to deal with anyway and not your work to do.

They are the only ones ready for battle and it is a false battle that we have all been programmed or led to believe that it is our job to judge.

It is not even your job to judge yourself. Awareness, my friend, is all we need, awareness of do I actually need to act here when opposed? Is it my job to get involved in other people's opinions and thoughts of me or is that their business?

So, sing on freely, sing on my friend, sing your tune. Sing it loud and sing it proud as they say. You never needed courage, you just needed your truth and to speak up, lovely one.

Rage

"Stay calm she says, stay calm. My waters are stirred up by the moon, tugging like a boat to the jetty. When the waters are wild at sea, the same way the wind is whipped up before rain as it forcibly makes its way down open streets with rage. Catch yourself if you can in stillness, seated in the storm, anchor to mother Earth for she has seen it all before. You are not the first and you won't be the last to feel this energy rising; stay calm she whispers, stay calm, until the tide is as silent as the dawn of a new day. Harness the energy and control it with ease like the sails on a boat in the stormiest of seas."

I feel I am a strong, fiery woman at times and in that, there are both feelings of power and strength and then shame as my fire runs wild and gets out of control becoming destructive at times (yes, I am woman).

For as long as I can remember, I have felt a strong drive and connection to a powerful force of rage surrounding justice (or injustice, should I say). Whenever I witness it, like a storm surge, emotion takes over from a primordial root source. I leap into action with a resurgence of energy triggered by a spark from below that usually results in many emotions and a vocalisation of justice. This has left me at times feeling both empowered and disempowered at the same time. Disempowered because I usually am quite reactive in such situations and seem yet to tame my inner she-wolf in a controlled manner that would see me more as a she-human. The feeling of empowerment is, of course, short lived and just a by-product of the strong energy coming up from my root chakra that clearly needs some healing (quite possibly generational). The wounded warrior needs reassurance of stability and justice in his/her world, and it is a reminder in times like these to send love and healing to this part of myself so that I may respond differently next time, and whilst injustice still may occur we don't need to carry all the wounds of the past, both collective ancestral wounds and our own. We also don't want to display this to the next generation who no doubt will carry their own set of warrior wounds from the past and certainly don't need to continue to witness ours through displays of rage.

A balance and controlling of energies along with healing in the root chakra can assist us with future healing of humanity. This is not to say you shouldn't speak up and speak out, but do it with control, almost as if the same energy was slowed down and the whole process could change its course. Bringing some cooling energy into a fiery situation could have a totally different outcome. It is in these moments for me that I know I have a long way to go. Collectively we have much healing to do that cannot be rushed but needs to be healed moment by moment through evolution, mindfulness, and a strengthening of our connection to each other.

chapter 12
embody soul love

"When we embody love, we are the most powerful being in the Universe."

EMMANUEL

A Way Back to Love – Finding Peace in Meditation

There is so much peace in silence: silence of the mountains, silence on a rainy day, silence at the end of a song. Sometimes we have to actually listen for silence in between the sounds. We can do this by moving our awareness from sound to sound and finding the silence in between. There is silence in stillness and peace surrounds it. Observe the stillness of a candle flame, a statue, or a rock. There is peace in the rain that falls from the sky and in the air that is light and dry. There is peace in a picture that is pleasant to the eye or a song that soothes the heart. Raindrops fall from leaf to leaf gently playing their own symphony. Sit in stillness, observe, see things you never saw before, find peace.

When you know how you look at nature, at the natural wonders of the world, you will know exactly who you are. When you feel into the experience of noticing the greatness of it all, it shall be reflected in the perceiving of oneself.

Be the change – leading by example.

"When the power of love overcomes the love of power, the world will know peace." - Jimi Hendrix

Unmasked Without Judgement

Why do I do what I do? Be in the writing space, that is. Is it my calling? Is it my purpose in life? Maybe. Mostly, though, it is to share what's in my heart. It is to give, to offer up, all that I am and all that I will be through this life. It is more of a devotion than anything. It is both my light and my dark on a page amongst all the colours that life throws at us, and life throws us some colours, that's for sure. I want you to know that all of it, everything we go through, is okay. It's okay because it's all meant to happen. None of it is neither right nor wrong. We may say some of it appears wrong but in actual fact we are here to experience it all. Colour it which way you will.

It is hard because we don't always like what we see, hear, smell, taste, touch, or feel but we are here to experience it all. Why must we mask this though? Why do we feel the inclination to just experience what feels right or good only? Why do we run from the struggle, try to numb it, or chase rainbows? I believe that our ego tries to protect us, and in over protecting, it seeks ways to shield us from our own pain and fear which are not healthy for our soul and not healthy for humanity as a whole. In all honesty and truth, this slows down our journey of evolution and inhibits the soul from being authentic and true to this life. The truth really will set you free, but it is courage that will give us our wings. Part of living our truth and opening our hearts is also being courageous enough to show to the world both your light and dark without casting judgement on yourself and therefore others.

One of the most courageous things you can do for yourself and humanity is showing your true colours every day of the week no matter what colours may be dimmed that day or which ones are glowing. To do this, we need to heal from the curse of judgement that may bring ill feelings like shame, embarrassment, or worthlessness. These can follow us around like dark clouds, preventing us from being who we truly are if we were unmasked without judgement.

So this really comes back to a self-love issue and one of self-assertion, selfassurance, and self-worth. Linked to this can be your self-esteem that can be shaken to the core by the society we live in, by the societies we have lived in for centuries and so tarnished by generations of unhealed pain from expectations placed upon us by whom? Other people with other agendas driven by their pain.

So, open your heart to yourself first every single day by being all of who you are in every way, and you will be opening the hearts of every other human you come into contact with. You will be helping to heal others as they are slowly being shown how to give themselves permission to shine or not and just be true to themselves. Thankfully our soul stays true to who we are and so as permeable as our soul is, it is really more solid than a diamond. It is always there waiting for us to uncover it.

Teaching and Learning

In my days of teaching yoga, as much as my students would learn about themselves from me through yoga, I would learn about me through teaching yoga to others so much more. Who you are is what you find out about yourself along this journey we call life. You want to know more about yourself? Get into a relationship with someone else. One of the fastest ways to remember not just your light - as I believe that really shines through when you are on your own - but your dark, or your unconscious parts of you waiting to come into the light, to transcend, can be shown up when we brush shoulders or encounter others. Like the waves that gently brush against rocks and change their shape slowly over time, we too change shape through our interactions with others. Perhaps we become more of who we really are on the outside.

chapter 13
embody soul speak

"I grow silent. Dear soul, you speak."

RUMI

A Voice for Your Soul Self

Now more than ever we must speak up. Life is now and we do not get another chance at this particular life. Time will continue to tick in our third dimensional world and this life as we know it will cease. I must have spent half my life not speaking up and whilst it may seem like a simple thing to do, I am still waking up to the reality that I have not and do not speak up in all areas of my life just yet. The more I am awoken to feeling or being silenced, the more I wonder what role I have been playing all my life and for whom.

I have been asleep to my true self although somehow known about her all along. It wasn't until I fell upon the concept of self-love that my eyes began to open to how much I have abandoned her in my life. I abandoned my true self and put on the costume of people pleaser. I thought to fit in, to be liked, to be accepted was the goal.

soul self

Why else would I have been born? Why else are any of us born, here on this Earth? Definitely not to run in a herd unless that fits in with why you are here, your purpose and your true self. If you are at all finding yourself in regular situations where your narrative seems to be different or alternative to others' narrative as has mine, you may well need a dose of more courage than others.

Chances are you were born with more of this gift or strength to support your true self here on Earth. The trick is to begin to use it.

If you do not speak up, how will others like you know where to find you? How will you unite with your soul brothers and sisters? After all, the purpose of being you is to be able to unite with collective like-minded souls so that you may carry out your work here on Earth together.

What your soul dances to, your voice can sing. In other words, what feels like a good fit on a vibrational level, your soul is waiting for you to speak those words loudly. It is only our human insecurities and fears of being judged, disliked, or rejected that holds us back. It's time to sing your song so that others can learn the words.

A Time to Erupt

Feel the fire in your belly, like a volcano swirling with each stir of your soul as you reawaken. There will be a time to erupt, perhaps many times. When you do, it will come with all your knowledge, intuition, and experience backed by the strength and free will of your soul.

There will come a time to share, a time to speak, when within your heart and soul, you know who you are, and you will feel like bursting.

"And the day came when the risk to remain tight in a bud was more painful than the risk it took to blossom."
- Anais Nin

That is when you know it is time to embody the expression of your soul by speaking your truth, sharing your wisdom, essentially embodying your soul self.

When you do erupt, it will not be like a volcano sporadically, but carefully channelled, conscious, purposeful, the best kind of communication. It will be authentic and soul fuelled because you will know exactly who you are and what it is you are here to bring to the surface.

Days When You Are Not You, Who Are You?

On the days when our soul shines through, it is easy to be you. On the days when it doesn't, we are not really being true to who we are. This is when we need to take time out alone to come back to the self. When you might notice feelings of sadness, frustration, anger even, they are tell-tale signs that your soul is not happy, that there are blockages to your joy, to your soul flying free to who it really wants you to be. There is much we can do about that and some days it won't take long. It might just take a stroll in the park, a sit in the sunshine or a creative pursuit. Other days there might be deeper work to do and a meditation or some journalling might be in order. Of course, life can throw some pretty serious issues our way and some professional support might be needed.

Do whatever it is that you need to heal so you can get back to allowing your soul to shine through like sunshine! It is why you are here amongst many lessons and teachings in life, not to mention love and joy and adventure your soul seeks to experience. We can get weighed and bogged down in so much of life's stuff that is not even ours to carry. It prevents us from living and creating a wonderful world for ourselves and the people around us. The most important reason for us to get back to who we are is so that we can embody who we truly are to continue to be the human expression of our soul as much as we can.

It all starts and ends with us, always. We are the beginning and the never ending of our whole universe. Nothing ends in this life until our last breath, and then it is just a doorway to the next journey, our next rite of passage, to experience yet more of our soul self.

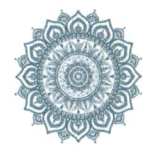

chapter 14
embody soul sees

"Intuition is really a sudden immersion of the soul into the universal current of life."

PAULO COELHO

Are You Listening? Intuition and Our Health

Recently, I began to experience strange sensations in my left leg, arm and generally the left side of my body. My first thoughts were, is this serious? Is this an impending heart attack, stroke or blood clot occurring? Having been thoroughly checked out and coming back to my senses I began to realise this was how my body was showing me signs of my own extreme stress.

It had been a period of go go go, new adjustments, a business, and a family illness to manage. It was a stage more recently that had not allowed for many breaks or personal life reflections. Whenever I would feel stressed or overwhelmed or anxious these feelings would come and then go when I had relaxed. For over 10 years now I had not experienced feelings like this in my body and the last time I did it resulted in an anxiety attack or what I like to call an unconscious, unaware release of mental and emotional stress that washed over me like a great tidal wave. It was something I could not ignore, something that finally had my full attention.

You see, when we push through, push away, or push down our feelings, trauma, or mental build up, it eventually manifests in disease of some kind. When we suppress, numb, or just don't have the space that we need to properly deal with our life's build ups, our body deals with it for us by bringing it to our attention in a way that we cannot ignore.

Your job is you, and as uniquely as you are built, so too will be your unique experience of life and how different things manifest, both desirable and undesirable. You see, life does not let any of us off the hook. We must all stop and slow down at some stage to face our challenges that we must overcome or pay attention to. We will need to see what we have not been seeing, to hear what we have not been hearing, to honour our soul and love ourselves unconditionally.

Sometimes this is just about taking time out, getting off the hamster wheel, and getting some real perspective on your life. It can be about reflection and the full moon is a great time to honour such a practice of stillness and reflection at this time as the month comes to a full cycle. In fact, the moon and its cycle of waxing and waning, full and new moons can help us align with our natural cycles and bring us back into balance. It can be a great indicator of how we can move with nature and ultimately the cycles of life the same way the seasons can help us align with our natural state as we interact with the essence of our physical bodies' nature. We forget we are nature; we forget we have natural rhythms like the animals and plants that are synced with the Earth. We are not robots, we are not technology, and we are not able to set a program that goes against our natural instincts and flow.

There are certainly those of us who are more sensitive to being pulled or pushed out of whack, those of us who are more sensitive to the world around us; nonetheless, this natural law applies to every man, woman, child, animal and plant on the planet.

If you believe it, astrology - the universe and the planets in our solar system - also can have a great effect on us. Just like the moon pulls on our tides and weather systems of the great mother Earth, so too do the planets around us affect our rhythms and flows of life.

So, are you listening, because the voice within is probably screaming at you by the time you get to the disease or out of balance state. I know mine does and the trick is to listen to the whispers. It could be a million different things for each of us; no two whispers are the same, for we are not the same. We are similar but never exactly the same and that is what makes us all so unique but connected at the same time. What is your whisper?

Please don't ignore it as your whisper is aligned with the very essence of who you are. Your whisper is your guidance system, your intuition, and your guardian angel. Your whisper is your bestie, and that bestie is you. You are the best friend you will ever have amongst all the amazing people and relationships in the world; the one with yourself is the most important. Trust yourself, trust your intuition, trust those gut feelings, trust the whispers however subtle. The mind may be loud, but your whispers will show you the way.

Contrast

The practice of meditation, tuning out, tuning in, or resonating with your own high vibrating soul in some other way such as through dance, music or other feel-good activities, is vital to continue to operate from the feel good soul that you are.

Just because you can't see something doesn't mean it's not there. If you light a match and burn some incense you would then notice the smoke float through the air. You would then see that the seemingly still air is behaving like ocean waves. The smoke seems to, whilst moving forwards towards the open window, rise and descend slowly and gently like waves on the ocean. In slow motion it mimics a whale moving up and down on the seas. You may never know about this unless you light a match to light the incense and sit quietly to observe this insightful phenomenon.

So, what does this mean, you might ask? Well, we don't know everything even by just looking with our own two eyes at what appears to lie before us. Sometimes we need to illuminate or draw on contrast to see what truly lies in front of us. Another example, phosphorescence algae can only be seen when its fear has been activated and at night. We wouldn't notice it floating in the ocean otherwise. Sometimes we need to go deeper than what the eyes would otherwise just see. Sometimes we need heat, a spark, or some kind of activation to truly notice miraculous things in our outside world and this also applies to our inside world.

On the inside that activation usually comes in the form of emotions but sometimes it can be other things such as physical pain. If we look at emotions, however, it is clear that some emotions feel desirable, such as joy, and others feel not so desirable, such as sadness. When we are confronted with the not-so-desirable emotions it is an illumination of needing to look deeper within and see what lies beneath the surface of these emotions.

Close the eyes and go deeper, engaging on that inner journey to remember the relevance and importance of what these emotions are trying to convey to us. If we begin to look at our emotions as being a miraculous phenomenon when they appear, instead of pushing these undesirable feelings away, we can see them as a blessing that our soul is telling us something is up and needs attention. Our soul will scream at us often when we are not on the right track or when we are not aligned with our core values and our true purpose.

The Observer at the Eye of Your Own Storm

Recently, I could feel waters stirring up inside me. The moon was pulling at my hormones and the rage like the quick wind down the street was brewing.

Coincidentally, there was a similar storm brewing outside with the weather. I was able to sit and observe the weather outside and the weather inside of me. From the lens of the observer, I also noticed a sudden stillness in the weather outside as if someone had just turned off the switch. It made me think of the eye of storms and I explained it to my children. As I was discussing it with them, I realised I too must have an eye of my own storm that I could anchor to or stay inside of and watch the storm around me.

In this way I was able to find a safe place to reside each time I felt pulled into my own storm. For the first time I was able to visually detach to the storm that was raging inside of me and notice it for what it was, a storm of emotions that would soon pass. I didn't have to be the emotions or the storm, I could just witness whilst staying in the eye and staying aware not to be pulled into the emotions. I could stay aware of the emotions, acknowledge them, notice them, and let them pass.

chapter 15
embody soul connect

"Embody the light of the divine being you are."
AUTHOR UNKNOWN

Masculine and Feminine Together

The moon has forever represented the feminine energies of the Earth and the sun the masculine. While the sun is hot and lights up our day for work or action and getting things done, the moon is cool, reflective and lights the way through the darkest of nights. These elements are one major example of the difference between masculine and feminine energies and there are many.

As I write this, today the moon is shining bright in the blue sky of the day. That's right, the moon in the day shining bright. Who would have thought? We may not see the moon until nightfall on most days but sometimes we can see her in the daylight when she is close enough to the Earth, in the morning or afternoon. The moon shines alongside the sun some days and together they are shining ever so bright.

Even though it is normally the sun's place to shine in the day, today the moon is present to the naked eye. When we embody the balance between masculine and feminine energies equally in our lives through the guidance of our own being and when we tune in, tap into our soul, we will find a harmonious balance of the two energies, no matter what sex or tendencies we may currently be or exhibit on the outside through our physical bodies. We are made up of both masculine and feminine energies equally and these energies are ours to be able to tap into and bring forth for balance in our own lives.

It is said that the right side of our bodies represents the masculine, and the left side represents the feminine, and when illness or injury occurs this can be a clue as to which energy might be pulling, pushing or in need of nurturing at the time.

These are times for reflection, meditation, intuition and tapping into your divine soul self for guidance. Everything has an energy to it since everything is vibration and we emit a certain frequency. Those energies can be masculine or feminine and usually have both components to them. It could be a song, a piece of art, a book, a plant, an animal, or a person. Literally everything will display a balance or sometimes imbalance of the masculine and feminine. One thing we can do is harness both these energies of our soul self and find the divine balance we need.

Oneness and Divinity

How do we embody oneness and divinity? Divinity is within us as our divine being and oneness is the connection we have with the intrinsic web of all life.

Understanding that everything is connected from a soul perspective and realising even though we might be separate physical beings, we are in fact one.

Divinity feels like home as it is the seed of our beginning and end, our pure essence. Like the infinity symbol, there is no end and no beginning.

How do we walk with this oneness and divinity within us in our daily lives? We achieve this by acknowledging a connection to all of life. By staying connected to our own spirit as much as we can. By embodying our soul self (aka our true self) in as many things as we do here on Earth and in our daily life. By staying aware of our true divinity and oneness, meaning this is in all beings, especially in those challenging times of conflict with others. We need to keep this awareness and rise above where possible when times are tough.

As Marianne Williamson says, 'It is our light, not our darkness that most frightens us' and I believe that it is still true for most people. We have been conditioned over centuries to fear our own light and our divinity and be blinded to our oneness and connection to each other and all things living.

When we are all able to fully embrace our divinity and embrace our connection to one another, when those days come more often for more of us, when we embody our soul connection, we will move closer to peace and love as we would have moved closer to our own light.

Walking With Grace

Assuming or embodying grace in times of struggle is the result of claiming our own calm, our own peace within.

There will be times when we cannot be calm or feel peaceful, when our waters are stirred up inside; that is a given. There will be moments where we are so deeply present in life itself that we forget to reflect or connect with our own divine being let alone remember we are all one. These times will be when we are most challenged by others or life itself.

These are also the times when it is most important to take time out to connect to our soul self. We always have the answers within, or above, should I say? In this way, and the more we take time to harness our soul self, the more we will be able to handle life and situations with grace and the more we will be able to walk each other home peacefully.

It is a journey. It takes healing, patience, persistence, and perseverance to achieve this more and more in your life but it is always worth it.

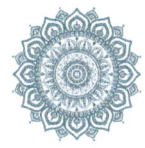

chapter 16
embody soul search

"With considerable soul searching, that to the utmost of my ability, I have let truth be the prejudice."

W. EUGENE SMITH

Standing in the Spotlight With Our Ego In Check

When I was completing my yoga teacher training back in 2014, I was afraid of what I saw as the spotlight, i.e., being the teacher up front with all eyes on me. It may sound silly to some coming from a grown adult, but the truth is, we have many parts to us that are grown in age but not in development. We stay stuck in our childhood fears of being judged, humiliated, or rejected by others when we are in the spotlight.

What I learnt was to let go of the ego that was ruling me and shift into the giver, to see that what I was delivering was a gift and of benefit to the receiver. I learned that this was not about me but about my students and the true purpose of me being there. Truth is it was straight from the heart and had never had anything to do with the ego so why start now I thought. It was so I could share this amazing practice that has helped me feel so good and I had always wanted that for others. I also learnt about people, in that when we are judging another, we are really projecting that self-judgement of ourselves. Of course, we may feel self-conscious for other reasons but whatever it is, if we dig deep enough, we will likely find our ego attached to all kinds of judgement in order to try and keep us safe. There is nothing wrong with judgement or being discerning in situations where we actually need to keep safe but most of the time, it's an overprotective ego. This keeps us stuck in a pattern of not being able to embody all of who we truly are and stand on the spot in our own light.

Rising Consciousness of our Imperfections

If you perceive yourself as a whole and fully functioning human being that is worthy of a voice and your own unique expression, you will not bat an eyelid when you notice your darkness rising or you see something in yourself that you perceive as less than perfect. Often, we perceive greatness or goodness as the goal in life, but the truth is it is only half of the human experience and it does not make us whole. In modern society we tend to honour the light on our journey and hide the dark attaching some sort of shame or guilt to it. There are valuable lessons in our darkness.

Sadly, we miss those lessons and opportunities for healing as we have been conditioned through society to push the darkness within us away, as if it is evil or should be condemned. Nothing within us need be condemned, just witnessed, overcome, and lessons learned. Since childhood there are so many situations as we come into this world that tell us we are not good enough, bring shame, unnecessary judgment, and generally steer us in the direction of having to be a perfect citizen, child, young adult, mum, dad, grandparent, you name it.

The truth is as Alanis Morissette once said in her song, 'No one's really got it all figured out just yet.' The other truth is, we are all brothers and sisters just walking each other home and as far as spiritual evolution goes 'No one is getting out of here until all of us get out of here' - Kaypacha Lescher. This notion implies we will all be coming back time and time again living many lives until we are all ready to rise together. We have many spiritual and karmic lessons to work through as a collective. Whenever you are helping someone else, you are really helping yourself and humanity rise as a whole.

"There is no coming to consciousness without pain. People will do anything, no matter how absurd, in order to avoid facing their own soul. One does not become enlightened by imagining figures of light, but by making the darkness conscious" – *Carl G. Jung*

Healing comes through 'shadow work' in the form of not suppressing your darkness but embracing it so you may be whole. When we allow our imperfections to rise, to come to the surface, we can see clearly what aligns with our soul, i.e. what is ours and what is not. Only then, can we go about shedding those layers, but not before embodying what looks like imperfection, what may look like mess and chaos and owning it first as our own.

Letting Go of the Need to Judge

Recently, I was tempted to unfollow a writer I had previously admired the work of. I had resonated so much with so many of his words and then one day I couldn't believe what was coming from him. In my opinion it was negative, judgemental, and downright raw and rude. I felt the darkness that he was in, and it was too much for me that particular day. Something in me refrained from unfollowing his work and I moved passed it. Weeks later, I started to love his work again and saw the light that was coming from him. It felt good and positive and uplifting and wise, just what I needed. I was glad I didn't unfollow him as I would have missed some important perspectives on life and humanity.

It reminded me to truly understand that we are all on our journey, this is our rite of passage and it is our virtue to show our true colours. If we continue to judge others on their darkness, we will never see the light ourselves. We all ride the waves of highs and lows with our lives and our emotions; some just choose to show it on the outside and some don't. I now thank him for sharing his darkness so openly as I was able to truly learn a valuable lesson. Our job is not to judge another's' darkness; our job is to witness our own. The most courageous thing we can do for another person is to hold space for their darkness, never to the detriment of ourselves, though, of course. I am grateful to him showing both sides as I too show many sides of me to the world. I have begun to care less about other people's judgements and know that my shadow offsets their light and vice versa. I know that my darkness, when it rises, gives permission to others to ride their wave and be themselves. We are whole and complete with our light and our dark and it is not ours to judge but to embrace.

"To bring peace to the Earth, strive to make your own life peaceful." - Unknown

Amongst us all lies a deep darkness that is waiting to be brought into the light.

It is both our destiny and our journey together to live out our collective unconscious karma that we have created in the past. Nothing is ever lost.

However, collective karma must be worked off through lifetimes of lessons and peaceful interactions with each other. If we truly seek harmony on this Earth together then we must begin with ourselves each and every day. We must consciously create positive deposits and actions of love, peace, justice, freedom, compassion, and understanding with open hearts and open minds every day.

'In order to create a peaceful world, you must create peace in your own life first.' As well, create peace amongst your relationships as much as you are able on your behalf.

You may be thinking to yourself at this point, well that's all great wisdom but is this really possible? In a world with so much doubt, disappointment and perceived failure, how can you really make a difference or really start to even see a difference in your own life by being your true authentic self, taking the societal mask off and daring to bare your soul?

We are but one light bulb in a myriad of lights and while this might seem impossible if others don't do the same, remember it only takes one spark to start a fire or one flame to light the way or one flame to light other wicks. Think about a chain reaction and think, what is the alternative? To turn the light off? Are you on or are you off?

part 3
shine

To Truly Embody Your Soul Self Is to Shine Your Light on the World

What does it mean to shine?

1. *(of the sun or another source of light) give out a bright light – Oxford Dictionary*

To shine is to live in accordance with your highest self, that is your true self. It is to live by your values, ideals, and beliefs and not live by another's. It is to not trade your authenticity for anything and to give out your innate gifts, qualities, and originality to the world.

chapter 17
shine soul deep

"I must be a mermaid; I have no fear of depths and a great fear of shallow living."

ANAIS NIN

Be Who You Are on the Inside on the Outside

What matters is that we can fully be our true selves. By true selves I don't mean the conditioned humans that we are on the outside but the incredible spirit beings that lie within us living in human form. The world needs you to be exactly who you are on the inside (aka that amazing light being that incarnated as you with all your true colours shining) on the outside.

Consequences of not feeling like you can be your true self and everything that goes along with that can lead to a painful existence and feeling like a flower that just never gets to bloom. A flower which is planted in an environment that does not support its growth is a tragedy.

Diving Deep

Often, looking deep within is where the water is crystal clear. It's on the outside that it is murky. We're often made to feel that looking within is only dark and scary, when in fact, at your pure essence level it shines the brightest. When we've dived deep enough to know this, we are never afraid to look within for we know beyond any pain, trauma or otherwise there is only light to greet us.

Your light greets you, the light which comes from its source, which leads to the realisation that you are not alone and come from the greatest light source itself and that that is within you. You are light source energy, and you are as powerful as that source. You are love and love has the ability to transform and transmute darkness. With this knowledge you can feel supported also knowing that love transcends all fear.

Any fear you feel about looking beneath the surface can only be met in the end by love, hence why fear is in essence an illusion and a mind made construct.

Imagine knowing now how it is safe to look within, as no matter what's down below, when you dive the deepest, it is where love will meet you. The deeper the dive, the deeper the love you experience.

Be fearless, dive deep, and find your shine!

'The world needs you to be all of who you truly are on the inside on the outside.'

Why Am I Here?

Once you have remembered your true self, questions of why you are here or what your soul's mission or purpose is in life may arise. We become curious about ourselves and the world around us. We are eager to know what our role is meant to be on Earth or what gifts and talents we might have to impart.

As I have stated in this book, I asked myself and others these types of questions when I was about 4 or 5 years old. I used to observe a lot and think a lot and I became the why child, pondering my own life and life itself.

Having some really good guidance and access to resources for these curiosities are necessary for a lot of people to explore things further. When I was about 18yo I attended one of my mother's yoga classes that she was teaching at the time. At the same age when I completed a pranic (energy) healing course, I really got started on my journey to understanding myself more deeply and the world around me more.

That aside I realise now that I have always had a close relationship with the self, as I 'felt' my way through life. Being an empath was my navigation system to what felt right or wrong to me. That didn't mean, however, that I always spoke up, but I somehow always just knew, and as I've grown I understand how important it is to just trust that knowing and trust what's deep within. It is where our shine comes from. The sun might shine down on us, but we shine from the inside out.

chapter 18
shine soul joy

"The joy we feel has little to do with the circumstances of our lives and everything to do with the focus of our lives."

RUSSELL M. NELSON

A Time to Shine

When will we rise? When will we stop hiding our incredible soul? When will we rest our heads and our hearts and let our soul in the driver's seat? What are we so afraid of? Who are we trying to please or what are we trying to prove by living our manufactured lives the way we're expected to? Again, why have we hidden in the shadows? Take the stage; this is your life. We all have our own stage. Get on yours; the time is now. No more waiting. You have the experience, life experience, knowledge, deep wisdom, deep knowing. You have all the materials, you know enough, you are enough.

Again, the time is now. The world needs you to be exactly who you are on the inside on the outside because who you are on the inside is who you came here to be, so be that. You don't have to settle for a mechanical human existence; there is so much more magic within you.

You can shine like the incredible human you were born to be because that is your birthright. Incarnate as your soul self, not as just an empty human vessel.

You are already full of life with that soul inside you; let your soul within shine outwards until you are so blinding to others, that others have no choice but to close their eyes and look within so they too can find their light. Maybe we are the torch that gets passed on. Be the torch. Be the brightest torch you can be or be a star or whatever you like; just shine bright. Your time is now so get ready to shine.

Joy as a Sign You Are in Alignment With Your Soul Self

Waking up joyful, for no real apparent reason, other than you just woke up that way. Perhaps after a really good sleep, with a spring in your step, when you notice the birds singing and the sun is shining through the clouds after the rain. Maybe it's an energy from the full moon or because the planets are aligned for you, but nothing really specific other than on particular days you are joyful without effort. So be it, be joyful, enjoy that your day is painted orange (a colour representative of joy) and get creative, connect with others, spread your joy, spread your love and light. Allow this energy to open your heart and propel you forward in the direction of your dreams. Use this energy to build upon your purpose and find strength in this. This is a time to focus on your hopes, dreams, and purpose! This is your internal energy signalling you to be your brilliant, amazing self. You become a conduit for creation of the highest order.

What You Focus on Grows

Whatever it is we focus on becomes our experience. Quite simply, if we afford ourselves the freedom to be able to choose what we focus on, we can choose things that inspire us, things that we are interested in and things that bring joy to our soul.

Even if we are in a position where we don't have as much freedom to do things that bring joy in our day-to-day lives, there are always the in-betweens. There's the pause at the end of a long deep breath, a 10-second focus on a beautiful flower, and an opportunity to marvel at the stars on a clear night sky or to appreciate things around us that interest or inspire us, that bring joy to our soul.

This can become a daily/nightly practice, like a meditation, until you begin to see the world through a new lens, until the world around you looks completely different from yesterday, just because you chose to focus on something in a new way, with every day as a new habit. Because what you focus on grows, so too did your joy. How much more joy could you bring into your day just by looking at the world in a different way, slowly, through the cracks in your timeline, like new flowers pushing up between the cracks in the pavement? Nature is doing it; we can too!

The flowers are like, 'Hey, I know this road is long but I'm going to be here in the cracks along the way because it's the in-betweens where the joy is found along the journey.'

Try and find three things that bring you joy each day, every day until it becomes part of the way you live your life. Big or small, it doesn't matter, just find three things every day if you can, then you will have a life filled with joy no matter the weather!

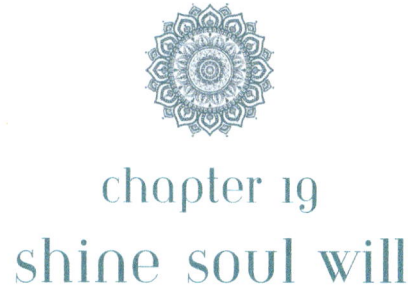

chapter 19
shine soul will

"The world will ask who you are, and if you do not know, the world will tell you."

C.G. JUNG

Being Comfortable

When we are comfortable, we feel safe to be ourselves. We feel safe around the people we have connected with, our close friends and for the most part our family. The more we trust and be our true selves, the more we give permission for others to do the same. In general, people appreciate your transparency, your honesty, and your openness. What happens though when someone we know around us disapproves of us in some way? Generally and sadly, we may close that part of ourselves off to that person and sometimes to everybody else. We can feel a range of emotions from shame to humility and may feel odd, weird, or different in some way. It can take great courage to be who we truly are around everyone, and it can also mean we are open to criticism, judgement or rejection.

So how do we be free to be our true selves whilst feeling safe, comfortable, and not fearing the world around us, because it seems like that could take some courage!

By now, hopefully these pages in this book have helped you in some way to guide you towards finding your courage and strength and have helped enable you to shine all your true colours and be your true self in spite of what others may think of you. Be so sure of who you are that you inspire the people around you to do the same. Hopefully up until now this book has taken you on your journey, allowing you to remember the parts of you that are unique and wonderful that may have been temporarily lost or shut down.

The truth is, we may continue to feel uncomfortable in certain situations. I believe these situations are only there to serve to remind us that we are having a moment that is not in alignment with our soul self. We are being reminded that this situation is not for us. In fact, you could say the more we are having uncomfortable moments the more we are waking up to who we truly are. There is a process at play here and it's leading you back home to yourself.

Going Your Own Way

Life will sometimes throw you some curveballs, some unexpected turbulence, some things that come from others you weren't quite expecting. Things seem just fine and then suddenly they are not. Sometimes we have to process and assimilate what just happened, what our own perspective is on the situation and what path we will take next. The most crucial part of it all is that you know who 'you are' separate from the situation and decide your path of action and stick to it no matter what the other person believes. This is all part of being in your own personal power, staying on the path that feels organic and right for you and going your own way.

It means not bending or overcompensating for someone else. Stay solid and true to yourself because that is why you are here, for your own journey, not another's. We are so used to being told in relationships to compromise and yet sometimes that can pull us off our own path and we don't remain in a state of being our true selves. I believe we can come to mutual agreements, arrangements, and understandings but compromising literally puts you in that compromising position. Why would you ever trade your soul for another? Why would you give your power away like that?

You can have a perfectly open, loving, and empathising heart and still put you first. Don't ever allow yourself to dull some of your glow that makes you sparkle and shine because of compromising. I would rather meet myself fully than meet someone halfway knowing that person too is only meeting me halfway. We overstretch ourselves and find resentment, dissatisfaction, and powerlessness in the long term and most of all not living our truth.

Setting boundaries is important. If I had never set any boundaries with my time, I would never have been able to write this book. I began writing this book during Victoria's second stage 3 & 4 lock downs in 2020. I have one high school child and two primary school children now at home 24/7 on top of what was five days a week of building an accommodation business with my husband.

Why now, you may ask, would I choose to write my first book in this time as well? The answer is I needed to connect with myself so deeply in such uncertain times once again and when I usually do that, wisdom in the form of words pours out of me and soothes my own soul, or rather my soul soothes me. Words and wisdom have always had a way of working through me, since I was a small child on my own pondering the world, to a troubled teen writing in journals as I listened to music, to a new mum in my twenties and through my thirties with the practice of yoga and journaling by my side.

So out of sheer respect for myself, my gifts, and my passions, especially as a mum with three children and having family responsibilities, I have to make time for myself.

Purpose

Sometimes we can feel on purpose when we are in action in our work in the world and other times, we can feel off track. We can feel like we are not productive enough when we are pulled by other responsibilities and things that need doing in our daily life that is not connected to our work. When these things pile up in life, as they often do, it is good to just take a pause. It is good to remember that every day counts in our life no matter what we are doing; as long as we are being our true selves, we are right on purpose. I'm someone who has three children all home schooling, a new puppy and a husband. I'm the mama and I'm often 'needed'. I'm also a very driven, purposeful soul who wants to do much work in the world and this pull can sometimes take its toll.

Today, I found comfort in these times when I cannot get to my work, that making sure I'm just being who I truly am in every situation can bring me some satisfaction, knowing that is my greatest purpose.

'My greatest purpose is to be who I truly am in the world no matter what I'm doing.'

For example, as long as I am truly speaking my truth when I interact with others, I am on purpose. My embodied work in the world is to be my true self with anyone I come into contact with throughout my day. No masking, soul self aware and just being exactly who I am.

chapter 20
shine soul love

"With an open heart is how the best things get done, the things worth doing, worthy and noble."

Living a Life You Love

Live a life according to your design, who you truly are and what you want despite what everyone else thinks or how society has been laid out so far. Find yourself, find your courage and develop the spirit you were born with to live a life that makes your soul dance! Remember your true colours, find ways to pave a new path and feel strong and unwavering while you do it. The Earth is your home as much as anyone's and although we have laws for good reasons to protect us, sometimes these can work against us when the expected norms of society clash with our own true values.

The pain and consequence of not living a life you love can be nothing short of traumatic and devastating and lead to chronic health issues and more.

My children inspire me daily. Currently my 8-year-old, who is sweet but fierce (in a good way), is refusing to 'do school'. She told me she wants to radically unschool (yes, she heard the term from me but no less than any other option that I openly tell my children is available). Why should they be stuck in a life they don't love any more than I or you or anyone should be?

All three of my children have been medically diagnosed as being on the autism spectrum. I think it's wonderful and my spiritual take on that is that they are here to create massive change that this world desperately needs. I believe they are born leaders in their own ways, and I will support them until my last breath to be happy and thriving in a life they love.

If I'm honest, from a young age I have always felt different, a little odd, the outsider, the observer. I have always been full of my own ideas about life and somehow run by my own deep inner knowing. As I grew up, I quickly realised how much of who I felt I was authentically, was not really accepted or had a place that quite fit here in this world at the time.

It has been a journey with my children in realising the apple has not fallen far from the tree and I want nothing but to fiercely support them and who they are to be their authentic selves. I am now to them the person I needed in the world when I was growing up and I couldn't be prouder to assist them in navigating and living lives they love that are in line with their true spirits.

Be the Light in the Dark

If we don't come back around to love, we cut off our own brilliance and power. We cut off our intelligence, creativity and light just when we are trying to get through the dark. We rob ourselves and our families of joy and life itself. We fail to be able to move forward with our greatest pursuits and therefore we are not serving anyone, much less ourselves. There is no progress or moving forward when we are in fight or flight mode. Whilst it is important to allow our darkness to have its time in the spotlight, it is equally important to allow for our light to shine once again. Be the beacon of light through the darkness and light up the world from the inside out. Share your love, share your beauty, share the juiciness that is you. We are here to bring love and bring light and never should we allow any guilt or shame from our past moments of when the darkness reigned in our lives to prevent us from sharing our light and our lessons of love with the world. At the end of the day, my hope is that these words will be more than just words of wisdom on a page in a book somewhere collecting dust on a shelf. I hope that I may inspire thought, that I may inspire action that will be remembered and rehearsed over and over so that my readers can embody their light.

Wild Open Hearts

With an open heart, always, have been my greatest moments, the moments where changes and breakthroughs happen, and life flows with ease.

This is the upside to an open heart and an open heart will always be one of my personal goals for this very reason and the fact that positive change comes when I'm in this state of flow.

I recall the earth literally moving from under my feet the year I trained to become a yoga teacher. Intensive training over 6 months saw my heart chakra and many others no doubt open immensely and the shifts in my life that year reflected that. The opportunities and doors that opened at the time seemed endless. Like I was floating on an upward travellator and reaching new heights everywhere I turned. I went from having to leave the property I'd been in for 6 years renting to owning my own home, from unemployed to running my own small business, from having an unreliable car to a car of my dreams at the time. Many other things were flowing it seemed and it felt like I was in alignment with not only my will, but divine will.

Mistake not, to have an open heart all the time is to be left vulnerable. These were lessons I would also learn after that time. Balance is always key. I left my heart on 'open' and there were some downsides to my always open heart. You can be vulnerable to manipulation, illusion, being used and eventually drained and burned out. I was giving, giving, giving all the time and not keeping anything for myself in reserve. I was a classic people pleaser. Looking back I needed some strong boundaries and to be more grounded. So, I am wiser.

Like a lotus flower, an open heart must dance with the light and the dark just as it does in nature through the day and through the night.

In this life a heart can never be fully open or closed all of the time and if it is, either way there will be consequences. As much as nature changes or transitions from one day to the next, the heart is just like nature and requires subtle changes in the way that is necessary to care for ourselves and for others.

You see you can not possibly have your heart open when the wild force of nature blows in the front door. It is too easy to get burned or carried away with the wind. The natural thing to do is to close your heart for protection and that is OK. We do not have to be hippy loving open hearted faeries all the time.

We are like the lotus. We even have seasons where we do not open at all and seasons where we are beautiful, brilliant and in full view. Nature can teach us so much.

When we are open and in a safe environment we can allow our hearts to be wild and free. The environment has to be right. The same for a seed to crack open and make it's way towards the light, if the conditions or the soil it's planted in are not right for it, it will not bloom. That is the same for us and our environment we are in, we must have the right conditions to open our hearts.

Of course it's life we are talking about and for most of us that takes some navigating as we may be in a busy work place, a toxic relationship or somewhere else that is just not conducive to opening. It is wise to keep our hearts to ourself in these conditions.

When it is safe however, oh how the sky is the limit. How we can run wild and free. That is how we are our best selves. We are designed to love and be loved. Just as the flower was intended to bloom so are our hearts.

It is our responsibility, first to ourselves and then to the world around us, where possible, to move ourselves to higher ground so to speak. When we are not in environments to run free with wild abandon, to create that space for ourselves in our lives.

To work through or remove ourselves from toxic situations. Not to stay with closed hearts but to run free with an open one.

The first step though is having an awareness about whether our hearts are open, closed or otherwise. To know at any one time what is going on with us so we can not only navigate and care for our hearts but move in an upward direction in our lives. Carried by our wild open hearts just as the wind carries seeds and spores to fertile ground so life can bloom again.

It's important to keep on the upward spiral in our lives and this is achievable if we remember to open our hearts at every opportunity we get.

Keep shining, keep rising, take care of your heart and it will take care of your life. It's intertwined with the universe and when you are open magic happens.

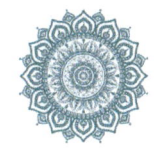

chapter 21
shine soul speak

"True power comes from standing in your own truth and walking your own path."

ELIZABETH GILBERT

Pathways to Truth

This can be a big one, a dusty one, one that requires shedding of many deep layers over time. Or, in fact, it can be quite simple. It can be as simple as meditation like using the one in this book.

Your unique self is the one who knows the truth, your truth, what's right and wrong for you and provides clarity on all the topics and questions you need answered and suddenly everything just begins to flow. You'll know the difference because this voice speaks with confidence, it does not ask questions or ponder, it knows the way and is like your best friend when, in fact, this is your brilliant self, not separate from you but always there waiting to guide you when you are ready to let go of your exterior world for a moment and go inwards.

soul self

These days we often find ourselves banding together with one group or another. 'Following' has even become a big part of our digital world.

I believe our job is to access our inner world and live that in our outside world; let it shine; let it lead; let it be seen. Let your truth shine through. Let there be no judgement and no attachment and let there be only love and brilliance, creativity and magnificence.

Daily meditation, you may hear that being recommended as much as daily exercise, good nutrition, and fresh air. It's certainly important to give yourself a moment and that's exactly what you will be doing, literally giving that inner voice a moment to be heard. It's so important if you want to live your life authentically as YOU, and what could be more important than that? Isn't that why we are here after all?

Creating the space on the outside to create the space on the inside has to be of utmost importance. We need to engage in an activity that brings joy to us so that we can begin to feel our soul. When we begin to feel our soul, we can begin to listen to our soul as it speaks and allow that guidance to become louder and the feeling of our own soul to envelop our whole self until we are that radiant shining light within on the outside. There we will find not only joy but boundless amounts of life, energy, vitality, and purpose. When we connect and engage in an activity that we love it sets our soul on fire and we become alive.

For me that is writing, yoga, dancing, singing, creating. There can be many activities and never has it been more important to honour ourselves, our whole selves, our whole entire beings by breathing life into ourselves and what we love. We must create the space and then claim our space with all that we are and all of our beauty that lies within.

Taking Up Space

We are so scared to shine our own light until we see others shining theirs. Only then do we feel we have permission to do so. What kind of a society are we living in where we fear our own brilliance, light, magnificence?

Can you imagine a world where we are not afraid to be our true selves, to let that soul self lead the way and just be amazing, every day in every way because we have permission, it's okay?

I have heard in Australia that we have a real issue with tall poppy syndrome. I wonder if this is the case in other parts of the world. There is nothing free about being kept down, hushed in society, or kept in line so as to not to make too much noise or steal the limelight.

Take up space. Expansion is what your soul wants for you. I know that's what my soul wants for me. Expand in every way you can, every direction.

There were things I would hear when I was younger that made me think twice before putting my hand up in class daring to say the answer to a question, show my best or be helpful. I would hear things like 'teacher's pet', 'goody goody two shoes', 'nobody likes a show off', and the list goes on. When it finally came to cross country running where it was encouraged to win the race, I felt comfortable enough to win and win I did. It became my thing right up until high school because it was an area encouraged and acceptable by the norm to do your best in without any ridicule.

I can honestly say as a sensitive child in the world, I had finally found something I was good at and relished in the challenge of doing my absolute best without feeling like a show off or the teachers pet. It was safe to take up space in this environment and so I did. How conditioned we can be.

A Life Lived in Full

Life doesn't always work out the way you want it to, it just doesn't, until you get clear about who you are and what you truly want and actively go about creating it. You need to dig below the layers, look back at who you were when you came to planet Earth as a soul, and evaluate whether you are living the life your soul intended to.

I often look to a childhood photo these days for inspiration. Can you believe it? Yes, I look to a child for inspiration. Sounds funny, doesn't it? Well, no, not really and I'll tell you why. That child staring back at me in the photo knows exactly who she is and what she wants. Yes, children actually know and then we go and tell them something else, like they can't be that or they're dreaming and so on.

This makes me so angry that we do this in this world, that we treat children like we know better. Maybe with some things (usually earthly practical things) we may know better, but we do not know what is best for children when it comes to their life path. They know best because they are so close to their higher being. They have spent less time on this planet. They have not been entirely worn down by society, yet.

We need to be so careful with our precious children because I bet they know what is better for us right now when they watch us run around chasing our tails. I bet they wonder what we are doing and why we just don't do what we want to do. Children push to do what they want to do all the time. Go them!

As I sit writing this, it is a public holiday. My two daughters, son and hubby are doing exactly what they want to right now at this moment and I am too, and it feels so lovely. I am sitting here spending some time with my inner soul and allowing her to tell me exactly what she wants. I'm listening to some very beautiful grounding, soulful yoga music; sipping delicious herbal tea with a candle lit and just flowing free on the keyboard with all that I am in this moment.

For me this is pure bliss. I feel like the reason it is pure bliss is because I am so close, right in alignment with my soul self right in this moment and I love her; I love who I am. I often say that the person, the fun, the adventure, the way I have been looking for is all within myself. There is an infinite universe within us.

There is never a need to look outside.

That said, we are here to create, to take up space, to be expansive, to exchange and to learn and to grow. Outside is to experience all that we are on the inside on the outside in pure physical form. So, bring you out, paint the world around you with your unique brush, leave a soul print on every corner of the world you touch, on every person you meet. You would have lived a life in full if you lived with everything that you are on the inside on the outside. You could never argue that your life was incomplete. Just be you in every moment. Speak up when you need to, go where you want to, create what feels good to you. Make it a life lived in full.

chapter 22
shine soul sees

"Follow intuition, for intuition is the magic path."
FLORENCE SCOVEL SHINN

What I Know for Sure

Oprah Winfrey once said, 'what I know for sure' and it really stood out to me; these five words said slowly had a tremendous impact on me and I felt it deep within my soul.

These five words are almost what this whole book, my whole life, and all of me stands for. These words reside deep within me, not taught on the surface, but what I know for sure, deep within my soul.

It's even more than intuition and definitely more than a hunch; it's so deeply certain and entwined within us, woven through us over lifetimes and lifetimes; it's our 'knowing', quite simply, but not to be brushed off or taken lightly. It's what we come here with and tend to forget in the noise of the world and then when we get older, off track or run into trouble, instinctively we try to uncover it. We know it's our saviour, has all the answers for us and is always there to catch us when we fall or when we are seeking answers, truth, or direction. Our soul's guidance comes to us through this deep knowing and what you may hear people speak of as intuition. It's available to all of us and will come to us and be accessed if we develop a relationship of trust, faith, and belief in ourselves.

So here is what I know for sure about the light and the dark. I know for sure that if you allow yourself to embrace the light, if you allow yourself to be brought into the light when the opportunity arises and completely one hundred percent immerse yourself, there you will find the light of your soul. Then from that point everything flows, deeply emersed in the brilliant light of who you truly are, within the magic woven tapestry of this world. You will light up, you will overflow with light, with love, with inspiration, with energy, with universal love. All your chakras will open up, you will flow, you will spill over, and the magnitude of who you are will become apparent not only to yourself but to the world around you as you touch and imprint your sparkle on every being, animal and part of this Earth that you come into contact with, that you meet.

What I know for sure is that the same is true for the darkness. It will kick you in the butt, it will pull you down so deeply if you allow it. Whatever you do, keep your head above the water. Immerse in the darkness but just keep your lips above the water so you can breathe, so that when the time comes, you can slowly draw yourself out from the darkness you have needed to be in. This is so you can be reborn into the light and reach higher highs than the lowest of lows that you've ever known. When you reach those highs, stay with that feeling, do whatever you can to keep that ball rolling.

They say make hay when the sun shines, but have you ever tried weaving baskets in the night under the stars? Don't stop weaving, don't stop creating, don't stop paddling beneath the surface until you are able to come back into the light. Be all that you are and don't stop. Uplift, uplift yourself, uplift this world, uplift the people around you, when you have the strength.

Send out love beyond measure because your time in the darkness will come once again. Like the rise and fall of the waves, the rise and fall of the sun, the rise and fall of the moon, and the rise and fall of the temperature, your time will come once again. Do your part while the love is lifting you high and reach out to people that need this energy. Send love to the world, do your part in a give and receive manner and when your time comes it will return to you in ways that will support you through your darkness or whatever colour you are riding through at the time. Life can run you ragged and, as you get older, unless you are plugged in, tapped into your own source that keeps you on track most of the time and bobbing above the surface, your resistance becomes less and less. This is more reason for your need to set boundaries and to strengthen your own resistance against putting up with things you don't need to. Stay pure, stay light, stay in the love to the best of your ability.

To find the light within you, you've got to shake off the feeling that you don't deserve the light or the love or abundance. You've got to feel like you deserve these things, set the stage, and tell it how it is. It doesn't matter what you've done in your past, your karma, parts of you, or if you wish you'd never acted in a certain way or done certain things. What matters is your future and what matters is now.

To transcend the darkness is our job. The light beings, the light bringers, the light givers help us transcend our own darkness. Often, we come here with the darkness to face, and it is up to us to rise above and overcome our adversities, our past, our own triggers, our own imperfections. It's up to us to let go, be calm, relax and know that most likely we will never completely achieve transcendence of all darkness in one life but to keep on rising anyway. To know that it is a collective pursuit and we are not alone on this mission.

Be a magnet and never stop believing that you deserve no matter the depths of the darkness that you face. Never stop believing in you, never stop believing that you deserve, that you can make it, that you can do it.

Be the leader, show the way, be the light and be the darkness, shine light on your darkness and shine light on your light. Be honest, be real, be raw, be open, be unafraid, be free, and be you.

Insights

'We are given many glimpses into who we truly are as we grow up. If our eyes are open enough, we will take note.'

When I was younger, my mother would scrunch her face up and say to me, 'Oh, you're so wise!' like it was sickening to her after I had said some sort of sentence about something. Unfortunately, I probably focused on her expression more than what I had actually said as it was a surprise to me that something that fell out of my mouth so naturally could yield such a response. No doubt, I'm sure she was secretly proud deep within that little person had shone her natural soul self and speak up without a care in the world. When did we learn to shut up, I wonder?

Never did I think that one day I would be an author, but perhaps if I'd listened more to me and less to the world around me, I may have arrived at that conclusion sooner. I do believe in divine timing, however.

There are many signs along the way that show who we truly are. We must let go of our heart and let go of our head to listen to our soul self.

Soul Perspective

Intuition without bias, as intuition is a clear vibration of truth, is like flying above and looking down to see everything from the clearest vantage point. We can rise above bias, false truths and trickery due to a vibrational frequency that literally emits a frequency of truth above anything else. It's a soul perspective, a clear one, straight from your higher self. It's one that's shining directly from your soul with no question about it. Trust it. This is your personal perspective from your soul self.

We may get goosebumps when talking about something to a friend that is our absolute truth, when we are waking up to a new truth, or some new perspective occurs to us for the first time that has cut through a once prior illusion. One thing is for sure after reading this book, if there is one person you trust, let it be you. Your light and your soul perspective are all you really need.

chapter 23
shine soul connect

"A strong soul shines after every storm."
AUTHOR UNKNOWN

Cycle of Life and the Infinity

If we never stop learning, then we never stop growing, and if growing can bring us pain, then perhaps we should never stop expecting pain because maybe when we are hurting, we are actually growing. Perhaps we are here to grow into our colours and as we grow through our darkness, each time our colours strengthen.

Perhaps all those rainbows in the sky we see on dark days are our ancestors reminding us to shine bright, not like the sun but like the rainbows that we are.

Instead of chasing the sun we should be chasing the rainbow. We will go round and round on the infinity train many times over until we have learnt all our lessons, completed all our tasks, and graduated into the school of light. We will continue to be given a glimpse of that light along the path of darkness to keep us focused on the light; however, it will be our true colours that fuel our journey into the heavens above. We must trust in the process; we must trust in the cycles of life and enjoy the journey. We are here to experience our infinity, our unique path and journey.

We never stop coming out of the dark into the light. It is not a straight line though; like the infinity symbol, we circle and loop back around on an endless journey of ups and downs, twists and turns. We go through the dark and we come out the other side over and over again. Like being caught up in a wave tumbling you to the shore, just when you think it won't end and you can't breathe, you wash up on the shore, not just once but multiple times, cycling through life or lifetimes. This is how strong you are, how many strings you have to your bow, how immortal your soul is. It happens not just throughout the one lifetime either, but throughout many lifetimes and across many timelines, dimensions, and galaxies.

Throughout this life we are not just the one butterfly, once, but we repeat the cycle many times in many different ways. We are dimensionless. There are many dimensions to us. We have many lessons to learn and many to teach. Have plans, but take it one day at a time, for each day is truly a gift.

Sacred Soul Self

If we are not being our sacred soul self, then who are we being? Now more than ever, it's so important to be who your soul truly is. That is what you came here to be. I believe when we achieve that fully (and I am in no way proclaiming that I, myself, am there fully as the journey can be long), we will achieve peace and love and have compassion, empathy, understanding, and all the things we need to inhabit to make the world go around collectively. We will achieve all the things that require us to work together as a human race, not tear each other apart.

Right now, it is my belief we are under a spiritual test, a test to see whether we will allow what may seem soft to some, our spiritual self, to rise above our human minds and ego self or allow the illusion of strength to continue to drown out our truest power, our soul self. I think this is the greatest test on our planet and one we have come here to realise. Perhaps that's what realisation of the soul means, to realise that our true self is the one with the true power, the true force, even the true immortality.

While we see millions try to outsmart 'life' by pouring copious amounts of money into technologies driven to extend life as we know it on a human level, reach the moon or find other planets to inhabit, perhaps that money would be better spent on true health for our bodies, minds, spirits and our given planet and animal friends so that we may enjoy quality of life here and now. We have what we are given.

There are so many technology 'seekers' these days, but what are they even seeking? Some fantasy world far away, some solution to the supposed problems we have now? Not one problem exists inside your soul; your soul is immortal, here and now and also forever. There is nothing to seek outside of this life for we are all of life in this present moment, and in this present moment is all of life itself.

Life is a true test of our faith, our faith in something greater than what the eye can see, the hands can touch, the skin can feel. It is a test to see if we can or will remember our sacred soul self and rise as that beautiful being, inhabit that self here on Earth and walk the planet and show the world our true colours, our true power, and our magnificent self.

The world is waiting for you; rise so you can help others rise. Find that light that is within you; never doubt it and let it guide you on your path, like the flow of a river guides a leaf out to sea. I will meet you there.

Standing Alone

The past few years, more than ever, I have had to stand quite alone. No doubt many others have also had this experience too with all the changes, divides and challenges we've faced globally. I now feel I am beginning to swim to the top, however, having found my place in the world, who I truly am and sacrificing no parts of me for the sake of anything else. I am too important and so are you! My soul is happy to say that I have learnt strength and true resilience and have a true grounded excitement for my future as I walk my path the way my soul intended.

One thing standing alone teaches you is your own inner strength and how whole you truly are. There is true freedom to be found within this and an inner peace that cannot be disturbed. It's like peace, love and freedom has become my holy trinity.

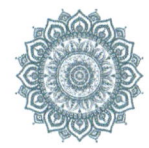

chapter 24
shine soul search

"In order for the light to shine so brightly, the darkness must be present."

FRANCIS BACON

Not Just Black and Light

Our imperfections, like the natural edges on a crystal or the wear and tear on a rock, become the perfect edges that, when the light shines on them, reveal brilliant colours that are made up of pure white light. Without the dark, our true colours could not be seen, for to see the true colours of the light it can only be seen after bouncing off an edge. When we allow the light to shine from our edges or our cracks, our colours are revealed so that we may see our true beauty.

There is the dark and light and all the colours in between. It's not all black and light but all colours of the rainbow that make up our real magic we hold inside.

When navigating the whims of life and diving into your dark, don't forget about the spectrum of colours that can be found when searching for the light. It is this spectrum that holds the diversity of our soul self, the one that makes us unique, the truth we have been looking for.

Rainbows of Light

With a background in teaching yoga and a knowledge and experience of the energetic chakras that resides in every living thing, I have organised my writing to the best of my abilities in alignment with the relevant area of life that pertains to each chakra that we have. The connection and the relationship between where we might struggle in life and where we might thrive can have a lot of bearing on whether our chakras are fully functioning in a way that is supportive to us or not.

The key is to strengthen, open, let light in all the chakras so that we may shine like the incredible humans that we have the ability to be. I have also, in my experience, drawn a correlation between both problems and solutions in my life existing due to an area of my energetic body components including the chakras being in a healthy state or not.

For example, you may find yourself with a sore throat when the creativity in you is being stifled. While there are no hard and fast rules, I have observed many times in my life the relationship between issue and body disease. The chakras are an energetic wheel that exists and can literally provide strength and vitality to your life when functioning well or be an indicator of an area of your life that needs attention.

Hopes for Humanity

It is my hope that one day we may live in a world where our unique, whole, authentic self is not just accepted but celebrated no matter the shadows, no matter the colours that are shining at the time or the ones that may be dimmed. I hope one day we may live in a world where we are aware enough to not inflict our dark upon others but instead bring it into the light with others through awareness, courage, wisdom, knowledge, strength, and grace. We are not only here to live but we are here to love, to lift each other up, to hold each other in times of darkness without judgement, attachment or alternative agendas. I believe we are here to walk each other home and while we are not yet perfect at this point in time of our 3D world's evolution, we are whole.

conclusion

As I write this book and reflect on my own life, it blows my mind how suppressed I have been, how much I have been afraid to be me. I've innately actually always 'known' my true self yet let her sit behind fear so that human me would never be faced with humiliation, rejection, judgement and so on. It is time to let her scream and shout and let it all out. I feel a great sadness for all the times in my life I was afraid. The adult in me says no more.

"Be the person you needed when you were younger." - Ayesha Siddiqi

Never again will I be afraid to speak my truth and if I am, I shall read my book all over again. Sometimes you just need to be reminded of why and how important it is to speak your truth, to be seen, to be heard and to be loved by yourself, for yourself and for others who may need to do the same.

It is my hope that this book will continue to bring you out of your shadows in every situation in your life, that you will not shy away and that you will know that you are worthy. Know that you are needed in the world because you are here. We all have so much to share, to give, and to impart on the world before we depart.

"A life lived in fear is a life half-lived." - Baz Luhrmann

Remember to spend some time in silence, in quiet, and alone daily if you can; it is how we hear ourselves clearly. Sometimes I think we are afraid of the silence not because of any darkness that may arise but because of our light, because when we hear who we are we consciously know we will be denying ourselves if we don't be ourselves.

"It is our light, not our darkness, that most frightens us." - Marianne Williamson

Finally, self-love is the greatest gift we can give ourselves that will, in turn, become our gift to the world. When we embark on the journey of self-love, we not only find ourselves, but we honour who we are. We find worthiness that ensures we bring ourselves out of the shadows and into the spotlight.

"The greatest tragedy of all is to spend a lifetime never truly embodying who we came here to be and leaving this Earth's plane bare of our innate magnificence."

Doing your greatest work in the world and walking your path you may find are a couple of the best ways to not only embody your soul self but begin to let it shine outwards. Most people barely scratch the surface of who their true selves are, so if you have stayed with me through this book and come this far, your soul self will be jumping for joy by now! Only when you find your path, through knowing yourself and embodying that being, will you come to shine your true light.

Yes, it takes work! It is far easier to turn a blind eye, stay in bed under the covers or ignore your inner being as we've probably been influenced to as we grew up in this world. It can feel like the world is against you at times, that you are the only one who believes in your dreams, but never forget your soul self. The universe has got your back all the way! The universe is a pretty powerful light, wisdom source, and energy source to have your back. It's literally out of this world, unless we embody it, of course, and bring its potence and magnificence into this world. That is your job.

Remember when all is said and done in the third dimension of this world, your inner being is very powerful. It is creative, wise, knowledgeable, thinks highly of itself, has no ego attached, knows no boundaries in a positive sense where expansion is the goal. Our job is to bring light to the planet; it comes to us to be worked through us. To think you can raise the vibration of planet Earth just by being your true self, how amazing is that?

You can effect change in the people close to you, around you and further away.

In fact, like a ripple effect, you are a drop in the ocean here on Earth and it can vibrate out through the entire universe. We are all energy effecting change throughout the entire universe, channels of light source in motion. That is our true power. Know it, Embody it, Shine it, Your Soul Self.

questions and answers with the author

Q) If I'm operating on a soul level what does that look like?

A) If you're operating on a soul level, you are in flow more often than not. You are embodying the highest version of yourself.

Q) Does it mean I won't face life problems?

A) No, life problems will always arise; it's how we grow and learn, remember silver linings. However, life for most of the time will just feel more in flow as you will be doing what you are called to do; you will be doing what you came here for if you are listening to that higher self part of you.

Q) Can we operate on a soul level all of the time?

A) Never say never for anybody but I dare say that would take some practice, soul growth and a decent amount of work to get you to that position in your life.

Q) Are you operating on a soul level all of the time?

A) (Laughs). Absolutely not! I'm working on it though and seeing progress so I couldn't ask for more. One foot in front of the other, life lesson after life lesson, soul growth after soul growth, steady motion in a certain direction not forgetting to live in the moment each day enjoying my life for what it is now.

Q) What's the most important tip you could share out of this book?

A) To stay connected with your true self by taking time out alone, remembering who you are through your passions or who you are not by listening to what your soul rejects (very important) and getting as close as possible to doing what you love or resonate with each day to keep your soul alive and shining that on the world.

Trust me, your soul will be happy if you at least just set foot in one thing to begin with that you love. If your life is totally jam packed with work and responsibilities (and that's assuming it's work that isn't a passion of yours and is done to meet your responsibilities only) then your soul will definitely have hibernated. You probably won't hear it speak much to you as you haven't given it the time of day. Your soul is basically like a house plant: if you water it, put it near fresh air and sunlight and maybe even honour it in all its glory from time to time, it will thrive. If you forget about it because you're too busy, it's going to eventually die or at least be looking pretty shabby and sad. Just like that plant came here to live, so did you!

Q) What happens if we ignore our soul's callings?

A) This is a pretty big one. Somehow there are people out there who manage to do this and survive or exist but is that really living? I have a very sensitive soul so fortunately for me there is no way I could do that. I'd go as far as saying my soul is so strong-willed that it makes me very uncomfortable when I'm not on track or honouring it to the best of my ability at any one time. It is painful at times but a blessing in disguise all the same.

Sometimes my soul needs peace because it's got something to say to me in private. You can bet I'm going to start feeling like I need some time to myself asap. What if my relationship feels a bit off or I'm not connected with the husband? My soul likes connection, and you can bet she's going to raise that desire with said husband. Energetic boundaries are being crossed by someone? You can bet my soul will feel that depletion and rise to refute that. Soul is sad because she's craving connection with other souls? You can bet I'll be organising a play date for her and so it goes on.

Listening is imperative to living a full life that your soul intended to. Remember this is who you truly are, and your human self is here to embody that light. That can sometimes come out as anger, sadness, or frustration, and that is why we have feelings. I believe it's all part of our soul triggering us to put things in place for our higher good and best soul outcomes whilst here on Earth. So, our pain is a trigger towards our pleasure. It's a series of buttons that will get pressed to activate us into motion, that steady motion that will keep us on track or steer us towards what our soul wants for us. It's all just about paying attention more often.

Q) What does life look like when we don't pay attention?

A) If we don't pay attention, we're going to be pretty upset people a lot of the time. This will continue over and over until we work towards giving our soul what it desires. We are the vehicle in which to allow our souls to ignite and live this life.

Q) How do we first 'ignite our soul'?

A) Simply by listening. It really and truly can be that simple. Listen and begin to slowly steer your ship, small thing by small thing, desire by desire, what you can control in the immediate term.

Q) What is the importance of finding our joy?

A) We are here for such a short time that it is our duty to find joy and live a fulfilled life as close to our soul's desires as possible.

Start with something small; you may need to think back to childhood or your younger years. Was it roller blading? Did you enjoy pottery that you made once? Maybe it was something you tried once, fell in love with and never tried again. You are never too old to find joy. Steady motion in our soul's desired direction is all we need to live a life as close to our soul's desires as possible. It's what we need to feel alive, feel joy, and shine the way our souls intended to.

acknowledgements

Thank you to my many mentors, family members, and friends, past and present, who have helped shape me into the person I am today, with both the hard lessons and the more pleasant ones.

Specifically, I would like to mention Sylvain Dureau, my husband, my rock, the one who never stops believing in me even when I sometimes do. You give me the courage, inspiration, and tenacity to keep going and to keep aiming for what I want despite anything else. Thank you. You are my person. I love you.

I would like to mention Emily Gowor, my publisher, mentor, and inspiration to never give up pursuing my dream of being a professional author and writer and an inspiration to many.

Thank you for your patience, flexibility, and encouragement always. You are the reason this book has made it to the shelves and why I am becoming visible in the writing space.

Impeccably grateful.

Thank you to Jo Worthy. You have taught me to go forth and not care what others think in life and in business and what it really means to flex my courage muscle. You have taught me about true self-love and raised my awareness about people pleasing. You have also been a genuine friend and been there through some of my tougher moments. Thank you.

Thank you to Julia Dyer, someone I am very proud to call a dear friend. You are that rare diamond who helps people with absolutely no agenda. Your generosity of your time, resources, friendship, and sunshine is endless. You are my long-time friend no matter where we are on this planet. So much love!

Thank you to Luanne Mareen for assisting me on my path to purpose and for igniting the flame of the goddess within and confirming what I already knew deep down inside through the wisdom I carry on my hands. Thank you!

To my soul sister Pascale Clarisse. You are very special to me. I feel we will circle through many lifetimes together. You also provide me with inspiration, sunshine, and an understanding, not only as a sister but a soul sister. Invaluable. Love you! We continue to circle and lift each other up.

To my parents and siblings, thank you for playing your part in my soul's journey and growth.

acknowledgements

There will always be a deep bond and love no doubt no matter what. These relationships can be some of the most challenging; we've had a big role to play in each other's lives with lessons and teachings and I thank you for them all, even the hardest ones.

To the people who are reading my book, to the many friends and colleagues who may have purchased this book to support me, I hope this supports you back in some way. To my readers who get something from this book that helps you grow, I hope it helps to change your life.

You are the sole reason for sharing my writing. I truly hope there has been as much value in reading it as there has been for me writing it. Stay true to you X

about the author

You may be wondering who I am. What qualifies me to say what I say? How do I know what I know? It's very simple, really. Everything I feel gets articulated to the best of my ability and put into words. Most of what I say is from feeling, intuition, my beliefs and values of course, life experience, my corner of life and past, even parallel and future, occurring lives if that's something you believe in.

My innate wisdom is true for me, but please remember this book has been written to remember what is true for you. So, if some parts don't resonate, that's okay, it's not meant for everyone. It may touch some and trigger others, but either way, I hope it's helpful in ultimately knowing who you are and who you are not. That's what this is all about.

My book is hopefully thought provoking and enough to set you on your journey of self remembering (if you are not already remembering), embodiment of who you truly are (again maybe you are already there) and living a life from your soul's seat. It is so important that we be who we truly are; it is why we truly came here.

For as long as I have known, up until just the last few years, I have not felt a true sense of connection to many people, places, or things on any deep level yet.

It has been fairly limited up until now.

Perhaps my time is coming and the more I allow myself to be in alignment with who I truly am, the more I may attract people, places, and things that resonate with my highest self. I believe this is part of our great journey to the self, through the self, and back to what surrounds us.

From a young age I never felt that connected to where I was geographically and even with the Earth on any deep level. I looked up at the stars at night and wondered what might be out there. I almost felt more connected to the sky. We lived near the sea for the most part of my early childhood and in the ocean is where I felt the most at home, but if I'm honest at night I would still look to the skies.

I never grew up with any strong cultural or religious background; my dad was from a strict Irish Catholic background and my mum was from the Church of England. Neither parent continued with either of those religions into their adulthood and so neither myself nor my siblings were brought up with any religion. For that I am eternally grateful as my mum thought we should grow up and choose our own way and path, religious or not. My path was left wide open in many ways.

about the author

I never had any pressure to follow any religion or be anything that my parents wanted me to be; in a sense I was free. With the door so wide open came freedom but sometimes overwhelm. It was kind of just left up to me, and whatever I seemed to naturally be good at is where I put my time and energy. The world really was my oyster, and the open seas are where I sailed my ship as I grew up.

We had some family here (one set of grandparents and three uncles) as my grandparents migrated to Australia in the 1970s and the rest of my family was in the UK and Ireland, some moving to France. So, born in Australia I lived here with my parents and two older siblings, one set of grandparents, three sets of uncles and aunties and some cousins. More uncles, aunties, cousins, great uncles, and aunties were overseas. Our family was split in two: my life was in Australia and I was an Australian being born here but my immediate roots were in Ireland and the UK. We travelled the world for one year, literally, when I was 4 turning 5 years old. We went to Asia and Europe and lived in England for half that time where I began school.

We then returned to Australia until I was 9 years old and then went back to England again until age 14 years. I honestly felt lost, displaced and not from anywhere. We then returned to Australia which is where I have been ever since with the odd holiday overseas. I feel I had somewhat of an unsettled childhood, never really anchoring down anywhere, and this pattern or feeling of not being able to 'settle' anywhere has stayed with me throughout my life as I now constantly move from place to place around Melbourne / Victoria with my own family, and in the heart of winter look to living in warmer places.

My husband and I even took a year travelling with our three children up the east coast of Australia in 2018, dreaming about living somewhere warmer. To this day, if I'm honest, I'm still not really settled and I long to be exploring and touring this Earth as I feel there is so much to see now that my eyes have been opened and I have been shaped by my childhood experiences.

My husband's family migrated to Australia when he was 10 years old from Mauritius and I sometimes talk about the possibilities of us living there or in Europe. We are nomads at heart, and I think this comes from a feeling of disconnection to our distant cultures since our families migrated to this land. We are a mixed bag in Australia, and I never really resonated with any one culture so fitting in with a particular group has never felt like something I was wanting to do.

I must admit I also seem to get bored easily and want to explore this planet and its diversity of people and learn about cultures and religions other than my own.

There does seem to be a strong pull in me that is drawn away from western culture. I've never really felt

about the author

much of a connection to that and wonder about past life influences when it comes to this. I so much more admire many other cultures and their ways of life, rich in family and cultural traditions. Perhaps it is because the depths of traditions are held within the heart and that is a way to the soul self.

soul self

"Our deepest fear is not that we are inadequate.
Our deepest fear is that
we are powerful beyond measure.
It is our light, not our darkness, that most frightens us.
We ask ourselves, who am I to be brilliant,
gorgeous, talented, fabulous?

Actually, who are you not to be?
Your playing small does not serve the world.
There is nothing enlightened about shrinking so that
other people won't feel insecure around you.
We are all meant to shine, as children do.
It is not just in some of us; it is in everyone.

And as we let our own light shine, we unconsciously
give other people permission to do the same.
As we are liberated from our own fear, our presence
automatically liberates others." - Marianne Williamson

www.ingramcontent.com/pod-product-compliance
Lightning Source LLC
Chambersburg PA
CBHW062046290426
44109CB00027B/2751